Every Woman's Pharmacy

A Guide to Safe Drug Use

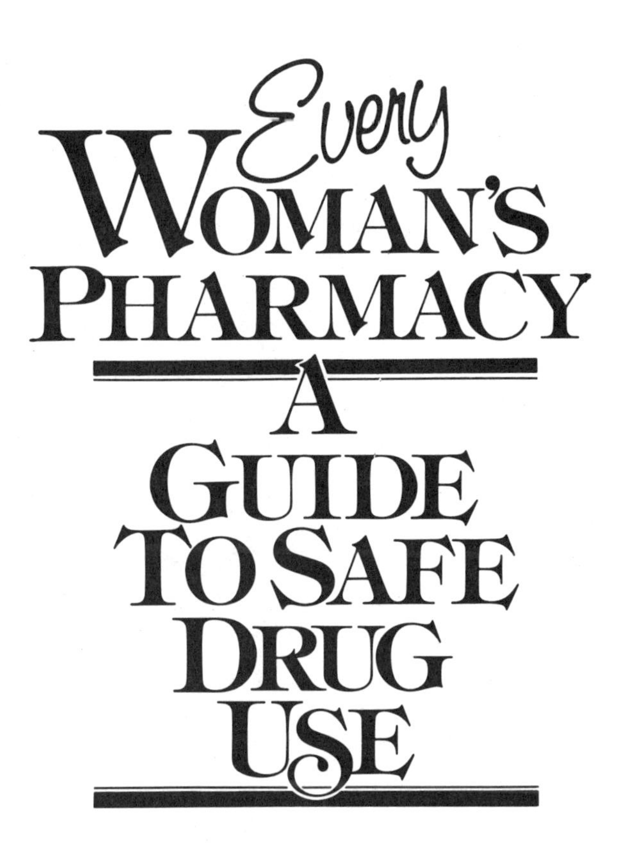

William F. Rayburn, M.D.
Director of Obstetrics and Associate Professor, Department of Obstetrics and Gynecology, University of Michigan Medical School, Ann Arbor, Michigan

Frederick P. Zuspan, M.D.
Professor and Chairman, Department of Obstetrics and Gynecology, Ohio State University College of Medicine, Columbus, Ohio

Jeanne Tashian Fitzgerald, M.A.
Medical writer and editor, Ann Arbor, Michigan

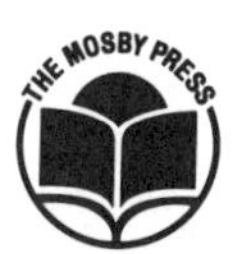

The C. V. Mosby Company

ST. LOUIS TORONTO 1983

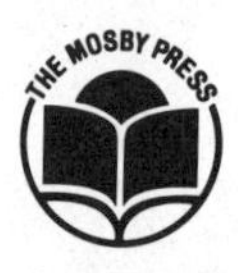

Publisher: Thomas A. Manning
Editor: Nancy L. Mullins
Book design: Nancy Steinmeyer
Cover design: Diane Beasley
Production: Barbara Merritt, Judy England, Ginny Douglas

Printed in the United States of America

The C.V. Mosby Company
11830 Westline Industrial Drive, St. Louis, Missouri 63146

Library of Congress Cataloging in Publication Data

Rayburn, William F.
Every woman's pharmacy.

Includes index.
1. Gynecologic drugs. 2. Obstetrical pharmacology.
I. Zuspan, Frederick P.
II. Fitzgerald, Jeanne Tashian.
III. Title.
RG131.R38 1983 615′.766 83-919
ISBN 0-8016-4030-X

F/VH/VH 9 8 7 6 5 4 3 2 1 02/A/232

To

Alanna

a continual source of inspiration, both inside and out

Preface

We live in a drug-oriented society, one in which a tremendous variety of drugs used for medical or recreational reasons is brought to public attention through the newspaper, radio, television, or displays in drugstores and supermarkets. Drugs used primarily or exclusively by women are plainly visible, but it is a bewildering, if not impossible, task for most people to keep up with currently available agents for menstrual irregularities, menopausal changes, sexually transmitted infections, infertility, personal hygiene, and treatment during pregnancy. Seeking advice from a friend, sales clerk, pharmacist, nurse, or physician has definite limitations. Clearly, there is a need for an authoritative reference for women—one written in an easy-to-understand manner. *Every Woman's Pharmacy: a Guide to Safe Drug Use* was written specifically for this purpose, so that the inquiring reader may become more aware of widely available and frequently prescribed medications—their active ingredients, standard dosages, side effects, hazards, and benefits—and to be better informed in choosing nonprescription drugs.

This book was written by two obstetrician-gynecologists and an experienced medical writer. Portions of the book are revisions of material from the medical textbook *Drug Therapy in Obstetrics and Gynecology,* which represents the combined efforts of 26 physicians and pharmacists.

Each chapter contains an overview of a specific clinical situation or disorder before discussing the appropriate drugs for treatment. The chapters provide examples of pertinent personal experiences and a capsule summary of "things to remember." Cost comparisons between generic and brand name drugs are presented in an appendix.

Every attempt has been made to present current and factual drug information. Our comments and recommendations derived from our readings in the medical journals and textbooks and from questions asked frequently by our patients. It is our hope that this desk-top reference will be helpful to you.

It would have been very difficult to write this book without the time, interest, and knowledge of several supportive persons. Pamela Rayburn, Laura Owens, Carole Karp, and Michael McKelvey were quite helpful in reviewing each chapter and in lending more insight about a woman's needs. Helen Hauck provided much assistance in typing and preparing the manuscript. Last, the many physicians and pharmacists listed below were active in writing chapters for the medical textbook *Drug Therapy in Obstetrics and Gynecology.* Some of their tables and comments were considered in writing this book.

Brian D. Andresen, Ph.D.
Gerald L. Cable, R.Ph.
William E. Copeland, Jr., M.D.
James K. Crane, M.D.
Donald M. DeDonato, M.D.
Jeffrey M. Dicke, M.D.
Chad I. Friedman, M.D.
Debra K. Gardner, R.Ph.
R. Michael Gendreau, M.D.
Paul E. Hafner, R.Ph.
Jay D. Iams, M.D.
Moon H. Kim, M.D.
Joseph J. Kryc, M.D.
Clifton J. Latiolais, Sc.D.
Peg F. McKnight, R.Ph.
Robert M. McNulty, Pharm. D.
Richard W. O'Shaughnessy, M.D.
Stephen F. Pariser
Randy F. Schad, M.S., R. Ph.
Philip J. Schneider, M.S., R.Ph.
Laurence E. Stempel, M.D.
Nichols Vorys, M.D.
Nicholas A. Votolato
Andrew L. Wilson, Pharm. D.
Kathryn J. Zuspan, M.D.

William F. Rayburn
Frederick P. Zuspan
Jeanne Tashian Fitzgerald

Contents

An Overview: Current Trends in Drug Use by Women

From the arrival of her first menstrual period, to the onset of her first pregnancy, to the final stages of her reproductive years, a woman watches with awe and amazement as the mysteries of her body unfold. The awesomeness has been intensified by scientific studies, which have illustrated the intricacies of the female reproductive system. Throughout a woman's life, one experience after another declares her femininity. Just before puberty mysterious changes take place in her body: tiny breasts bud, curves and new depositions of fat appear, pubic and other body hair begins to grow, and strange things happen to her skin. There is excitement at the first menstruation, which signals the beginning of fertility. Sexual activity follows, along with the responsibilities of planning or preventing conception. Pregnancy changes a woman's life with incredible force, be it deeply desired, unwanted, or unattainable. Abortion, infertility, illnesses, and imbalances of her reproductive organs all can make a huge difference in both the direction and quality of a woman's existence. Menopause signals that the rhythms and anxieties of the fertile years are coming to a halt; finally, the postmenopausal years present their own special set of issues, such as the continuation of sexual activity, a sense of lost femininity, and the fears associated with aging.

Accompanying these life changes are the methods a woman uses to manage them, and chief among these is the use of drugs. Today more than ever, drugs permeate our society, and their use is increasing rather than decreasing, so much so that people may have lost sight at times of what a drug actually is. Caffeine, alcohol, tobacco, and vitamins are used so routinely that we seldom bother to consider that they, too, are drugs and in certain contexts may be very potent. Marijuana, diet pills, and birth control pills are widely used by women. One study of many pregnant women found that they were the three drug types most commonly being taken at the time of conception. Tranquilizers and mood-altering drugs appear very frequently on prescriptions written for women, and women use alcohol at least as often as they use tranquilizers, perhaps more because it is so accessible. Without question, being slim and calm are among the goals of the American woman.

This book is about drugs—a wide variety of drugs—and a woman's body. No areas of medicine have received more exposure by the media than obstetrics and gynecology, the two concerned with the female reproductive system. An afternoon's worth of television, a monthly issue of a women's magazine, or the Sunday *New York Times* invariably produces an obstetrical or gynecological topic of some sort. It is certainly a popular subject of daytime soap opera. With this much information floating around, women deserve an accurate and reliable reference with which to make comparisons. This book concerns itself with the physical occurrences that are unique to women, the needs they have that can be met by drugs, the hazards of drugs in particular contexts (like pregnancy or contraception), and what they must know to make good judgments about drug usage. In addition to pregnancy and contraception, drugs used for menopausal symptoms, hormonal imbalances, infertility, menstrual discomfort, infections of the reproductive tract (including veneral diseases), and feminine hygiene are examined.

Every Woman's Pharmacy is intended to raise a woman's awareness of how drugs used for either particular medical conditions or for nonmedical purposes may affect their reproductive lives. It is about choices they have, and it provides guidelines to assist in making these choices. It attempts to reassure women that they can carry through a pregnancy and take the steps necessary to ensure their own good health without fear of harming their unborn baby.

Pregnancy is a consuming and undeniable experience; one can never be just slightly pregnant. The woman who has just learned she is pregnant finds it to be one of the most exciting yet confusing moments of her life. A multitude of thoughts race through her head all at once: Can it really be true? Will it be a boy or a girl? How will it change my life? Will it be healthy? Will I have a safe pregnancy? Soon after, the realization dawns that the pregnancy may be 6, 8, or perhaps 10 weeks along, and she was not even aware of its existence. The mother-to-be takes a look at the recent history of her life. She wonders if she's been doing the right things, like eating well and getting enough rest. She worries about any recent illnesses. She wonders if she's done anything she shouldn't have, such as had an X-ray examination or taken some substance into her body, a drug for instance.

Chances are quite high that she has indeed consumed something that falls under the broad umbrella of the term *drug,* whether it be prescribed by her doctor, bought at the local supermarket, or obtained from a friend for recreational purposes. A drug-free pregnancy is ideal, and if it is comfortable for a woman to complete her term without drug use, she should do so. Studies show that women are taking fewer drugs during pregnancy now than prior to 1978, possibly because public awareness about harm to the unborn baby and its connection with drug-taking is higher than it was 5 years ago. However, about 90% of women still feel the need to take some drugs during their pregnancy in addition to their prenatal vitamin supplements. The medications most often taken during pregnancy are vitamins or iron pills, mild analgesics like aspirin or acetaminophen (Tylenol, Datril), antiemetics (drugs used to control nausea or vomiting), antibiotics for respiratory or urinary tract infections, and nasal decongestants. Almost half the drugs used are over-the-counter rather than prescribed medications. Only a small number of drugs clearly harm an unborn baby, and these account for no more than 5% of all recorded birth defects. Hereditary and environmental factors cause another 30%. In the remaining 65% of birth defects, physicians and researchers simply don't know what the cause is. Evidence exists that certain drugs have something to do with birth defects, but more research and studies are needed. What are the specific effects and hazards of drugs most commonly taken during pregnancy? Which drugs cross the placenta (afterbirth) between the mother and fetus? Which drugs have been clearly associated with birth defects? Is a drug really safe if there have been no reports of birth defects associated with it? The facts need to be sorted from the assumptions, and these questions are addressed in chapters ahead.

Breast-feeding is more popular now than it was even 10 years ago. Nearly half of all new mothers breast-feed their babies, and there is a renewed interest in the benefits of this natural form of infant nutrition. Along with this interest is a concern about the drugs and chemicals that may get into breast milk and affect the infant. Many of the same rules that apply in pregnancy also apply with breast-feeding. Drugs used to treat specific medical conditions of the mother must be considered on an individual basis, and information about these drugs appears in the chapters on medical disorders during pregnancy and on breast-feeding. Some drugs appear in higher levels in breast milk than in the mother's blood, whereas others do not even reach the milk. Most of the time the benefits of breast-feeding outweigh the potential harm that may result from drug-taking.

Women have a wider choice of birth control methods available to them than ever before. With many choices, however, can come confusion. A good example is the controversy over birth control pills (oral contraceptives). Much has been said and written about them since they appeared on the market in 1960, some of it very emotional in tone. A few facts are clear. Aside from sterilization, oral contraceptives are the most reliable form of contraception available to women to date, when used correctly. Certain factors, such as high blood pressure, overweight, smoking, a history of blood clots, especially if found in a woman age 35 or over, add risk to the taking of oral contraceptives. Symptoms such as nausea, water retention, weight gain, breast swelling, and depression have been associated with their use. Pills available today contain a lower dosage of estrogen than did early brands, so problems have diminished considerably. In addition to being very reliable, the pill can have some beneficial side effects. Women using it often have more regular menstrual cycles, less blood loss and anemia, and fewer cramps. The pill offers some protection from ovarian cyst formation, ovarian and uterine cancer, cysts in the breast, and endometriosis.

Vaginal contraceptives do not alter the body or its hormone balance. They create a barrier between the sperm and egg but they do not have the track record of either birth control pills or IUDs. In actual use vaginal contraceptives have a 78% effectiveness rate in preventing pregnancy; birth control pills are 96% effective and IUDs are 95% effective. In addition to a high failure rate, vaginal contraceptives are occasionally associated with irritations in the vagina.

A basic concern of most couples today is controlling fertility, that is, preventing pregnancy until it is wanted (if ever). But 15% of couples have the opposite problem—infertility, or the inability to conceive when they wish to do so. Approximately half the incidences of infertility involve reproductive problems in the woman. Great strides have been made in correcting these problems, and at least 50% of infertile women who seek treatment can become pregnant with the assistance of modern methods of drug therapy. Even though these reversals of infertility are sometimes temporary and take a great deal of work, being able to produce a child is so deeply desired by some couples that any amount of manipulation can be tolerated.

Menstrual discomfort has plagued women through the ages, and although the term is heard less today than it used to be, "the curse" still seems an apt label to some. Many women are very uncomfortable during their menstrual periods, and the loss of productive time at work, at home, and in the community is enormous. The toll taken in the anxious days before a period must be considered also. In recent years, researchers have identified a body chemical related to menstrual distress, the prostaglandins, which are found in menstrual fluids and other tissues. Prostaglandins have a powerful effect on uterine contractions (which cause cramps) and hormone balances. Several new drugs that lower prostaglandin levels are now available, and they have brought relief to many sufferers of menstrual distress. Over-the-counter drugs advertised for relief of menstrual discomforts offer only temporary and partial help for the most part. They contain mild pain killers or stimulants, like caffeine, which acts as a diuretic (increases urination).

The herpes simplex virus II, better known as just plain herpes, has received a great deal of attention lately. This highly contagious and often painful infection has apparently reached epidemic proportions in the United States, especially among young people. In 1982 acyclovir, a drug to treat herpes, appeared on the market; evaluation of its usage and effectiveness is made in the chapter dealing with reproductive tract infections. Other common diseases such as gonorrhea, chlamydial infections, salpingitis (inflammation of the uterine tubes), and nonspecific urethritis (inflammation of the large tube that carries urine out from the bladder) and their recommended treatment are covered in the same chapter.

Feminine hygiene products are a big business. Somewhere along the way, the idea that the natural odors and secretions of a woman should be masked resulted in an array of consumer products. Naturally, every woman should be able to choose whether she wants to use sprays and douches to feel more comfortable. She should know that the medical value of most feminine products is nil, and they may produce side effects. Itching, irritation, and infection all have been known to result from sprays and douches. Douches can temporarily hide infections, allowing them to grow worse before a doctor finally treats them.

Until recently it was believed that a woman had to put up with menopause, and there were implications that it was mostly "psychological" anyway. Estrogen replacement therapy is now recognized as both effective and necessary for many women as they go through menopause. It greatly relieves hot flashes, sweats, and vaginal drying in many cases, so the transition into midlife no longer has to include discomfort and embarrassment. Estrogen replacement is associated with a higher incidence of cancer of the lining of the uterus (endometrial carcinoma) when therapy is not supervised and not counteracted by progesterone, the other major female hormone.

One appendix offers a comparison of costs for commonly prescribed drugs. Large price differences occur between drugs that seem to do a similar job for the same disease. There is also a difference in price between generic drugs and those which bear brand names. Because of recent legislation, consumers can request a generic drug when they present a prescription to the pharmacist and can often save money. Doctors are sometimes willing to prescribe the generic brand. Mysterious price differences occur from one brand name to the next, even though the drug is the same. The tables in this chapter enable readers to compare and learn who sells what for how much.

1 Nutrition, Diet Supplements, and Nausea Medications During Pregnancy

Most pregnant women spend a lot of time thinking about food. Besides being hungry, the informed and aware pregnant women of today know the importance of eating well during those very special 9 months. Some find food even more attractive than when they weren't pregnant, and their fantasies turn to thoughts of edible treats such as ice cream sundaes, pizza, salads, vegetable casseroles, cherry tarts, and egg rolls. Others find that their eating habits become eccentric, and they crave things like peanut butter and jelly sandwiches for 9 months. Still others, an unfortunate but substantial minority, find that food isn't appealing at all. Each meal is force-fed only because they know that the baby needs it and that food eaten by the mother is transferred in part to the unborn child.

Diet and nutrition

Obstetricians all know and emphasize the importance of a good diet during pregnancy. Whatever the mother's cravings, her diet must contain plenty of protein-rich foods, such as meat, fish, eggs, dairy products, brewer's yeast, nuts, and beans. She should consume a variety of fresh fruits and vegetables, and she needs whole grains such as bran and wheat germ, which can be found in breads, cereals, and waffles. Women should not be on weight-loss programs while they are pregnant, even if they are not at their ideal weight. Obese pregnant women should keep their present weight—and may even safely gain up to 40 pounds. They should concentrate on reducing *after* the baby is born. All pregnant women should avoid the well-known "junk" foods, like soda pop, candy bars, and greasy french fries. It is not necessary to restrict salt intake while pregnant, and it is undesirable to use diuretics to create fluid weight loss. Four or five light, nutritious meals spread throughout the course of the day work well for pregnant women, who may have an excellent appetite but not as much space for food, since the baby takes up more and more room in the abdomen as it grows.

A sensible, regular exercise program should be maintained along with a good diet. Activities like walking, swimming, and biking are all very beneficial to a pregnant woman, provided that she does not strain herself or become too breathless while performing them. The best advice is do what you did before pregnancy, but don't start new exercise activities during pregnancy.

Expectant mothers should be good to themselves and can enjoy a few indulgences like ice cream cones at midnight or lazy weekend mornings in bed with the newspaper. On the other hand, spoiling themselves must be done in such a way that it's good for the baby also. The single best habit to cultivate is 1 to 2 hours of bed rest, while lying on the side, each day.

Habits like smoking, alcohol and caffeine consumption (from coffee, tea, chocolate, and cola drinks), and using over-the-counter drugs should be kept to a bare minimum if they continue to be practiced at all. Excessive use of alcohol, tobacco, marijuana, and several other recreational drugs may have detrimental effects on the fetus.

A prospective mother should keep in mind that her diet is the one aspect of her pregnancy over which she has the most personal control. That diet is one of the most important aspects of prenatal care should be reemphasized. Mothers can derive great satisfaction from knowing they were responsible for eating the nutritious food that helped make their babies beautiful and healthy.

Diet supplements

The value of vitamin supplements is debatable. Certain people, like the well-known but controversial nutritionist, Adelle

Davis, have insisted that pregnant women must take an enormous quantity of food supplements to produce a healthy child. Others say that the average American diet is perfectly adequate and no extra vitamins are necessary. Most obstetricians fall somewhere in between, agreeing that some vitamin and mineral supplementation must take place, even in the face of an exemplary diet, but that excessive vitamin usage is both unnecessary and undesirable.

Iron

Pregnant women need significant amounts of iron for additional red blood cell production; otherwise anemia, easy fatigability, or weakness in late pregnancy and after delivery may occur. Normally, blood volume is about 4 liters (about 5 quarts); during pregnancy a mother's blood volume expands to almost 6 liters, nearly a 40% increase. The fetus, the placenta, and the umbilical cord all demand quantities of iron-rich blood. Iron deficiency anemia is the most common medical problem found during pregnancy. It occurs in 60% of pregnant women if they do not take supplementary iron and accounts for 97% of the anemias diagnosed in pregnancy. Even if she eats iron-rich foods or takes iron supplements, a woman will benefit from only about 10% of the iron she swallows, since not all of it is elemental iron, which can be easily absorbed by the digestive system.

One of the first recommendations an obstetrician will make to a pregnant patient is to have a blood count to determine the adequacy of her present iron levels. If a woman starts her pregnancy in a nonanemic state, she will probably not need iron supplementation until her fourth month. However, if she is somewhat anemic, she will need to begin taking in at least 30 mg of supplementary elemental iron per day immediately. Table 1-1 lists several prenatal and over-the-counter vitamin preparations with their iron and folic acid content. Note the wide variation between pills in amounts of both substances. Many over-the-counter vitamin pills contain no iron or folic acid (another substance that is crucial to red blood cell formation during pregnancy) and are not suitable for pregnant women. If you have a question, consult a physician; however, by the fourth month of pregnancy all women should be taking 20 mg of supplementary iron per day.

Unfortunately not all people tolerate iron pills well. They can cause nausea, gas, diarrhea, or constipation. Occasionally they

Table 1-1 Common prenatal and over-the-counter (OTC) vitamins

Trade name	Elemental iron content (mg)*	Folic acid content (mg)†
Prenatal vitamins		
Filibon‡	18	0.4
Filibon F.A.	45	1
Filibon Forte	45	1
Materna 1•60	60	1
Natabec‡	30	0.8
Natabec Rx‡	30	1
Natabec F.A.‡	45	0.8
Natalins‡	30	0.8
Natalins Rx	60	1
Pramilet FA	40	1
Stuart Prenatal‡	60	0.8
Stuart Prenatal with Folic Acid	65	0.3
Stuartnatal 1 + 1	65	1
OTC vitamins for general use		
Dayalets Plus Iron	18	0.4
Mi-Cebrin	15	0
One-A-Day	0	0.4
One-A-Day Plus Iron	18	0.4
Stresstabs 600 with Iron	27	0.4
Theragran-M	12	0
Theragran Hematinic	67	0.33

*Minimum daily requirement of absorbed elemental iron during pregnancy and lactation is 4 mg. However, approximately 10% of elemental iron is absorbed.
†Minimum daily requirement of absorbed folic acid during pregnancy and lactation is 0.8 mg.
‡OTC prenatal vitamins.

give the stools the color and consistency of tar, which a woman might mistake for blood. Taking iron pills after meals may help prevent some of these side effects, but less iron is absorbed at this time. Some iron pills contain a stool softener that counteracts their constipating effects. Certain preparations of vitamin C taken along with iron improve its absorption. Antacids should not be taken at the same time as iron pills because they hinder absorption of the iron.

Physicians sometimes find that their pregnant patients remain anemic even if they have prescribed iron. The main reasons for this are:

1. Patients did not take the pills in the manner prescribed.
2. Patients could not tolerate or absorb the iron.

3. The particular iron preparation used could not be absorbed well by the body.
4. Antacids were taken along with the iron pills.
5. Patients had an intestinal infection, inflammation, or growth that hindered the body's absorption of iron.
6. Undetected bleeding had occurred somewhere in the body.
7. Patients had another type of anemia that was unrelated to iron deficiency.

Women who have uncomfortable side effects from iron pills or who don't properly absorb oral iron can receive iron injections or even intravenous iron (if they are very thin and cannot tolerate injections).

An overdose of iron can be fatal; every year in the United States many children die from eating iron pills. Iron pills look like candy and often have a mildly sweet coating. As few as four or five high-dose iron pills have been known to kill a small child. They must be regarded as dangerous drugs in homes with small children and kept out of reach in soundly childproof bottles.

Folic acid

Pregnant women should see that they get adequate folic acid in their diets to aid red blood cell production. Folic acid deficiency is another leading cause of anemia during pregnancy. Recommended prenatal vitamins (as shown in Table 1-1) have adequate amounts of folic acid, and a balanced diet with plenty of green and leafy vegetables combined with the vitamin supplement should supply the pregnant woman with her necessary folic acid. About twice as much folic acid is needed during pregnancy as is normally required (0.8 mg versus 0.4 mg). Women who must take medications to prevent epileptic seizures will need extra folic acid during pregnancy.

Calcium

Calcium is important during pregnancy, and mothers should be able to obtain it in a diet containing milk, cheese, yogurt, or ice cream. Unfortunately, milk and other dairy products do not agree with all adults, including pregnant women. Bloating, excess gas, and abdominal cramps can occur after eating dairy products. Lactase, an enzyme found in the intestinal tract, is necessary to break down lactose, the natural sugar in milk, and lactase production tends to decline as people get older. Seventy percent of people of black, Asian, Mediterranean, Jewish, southern and central European, and native American origin have a lactase deficiency. In fact, it is the normal condition of the vast majority of the world's adult population. Most people of northern European extraction seem to be able to continue to drink milk successfully in adulthood.

Lactose intolerance is sometimes a matter of degree, that is, a woman may be able to drink 2 cups of milk a day (more than 60% of the daily calcium requirement) but will get sick after drinking 3 or 4 cups. Other foods that are not dairy products contain substantial calcium, such as sardines, canned mackerel and salmon, broccoli, collard, turnip, mustard, and especially dandelion greens, sesame seeds,and torula yeast.

We do not recommend calcium pills or supplements during pregnancy if milk or other suggested foods are consumed along with prenatal vitamins. The body makes adjustments during pregnancy that allow it to better absorb calcium; unlike iron, the calcium taken into your body is used rather efficiently. The old myth, "one tooth per child," can be laid to rest because the fetus takes only about 2.5% of the circulating calcium in the mother to make its bones and teeth.

In a few women with digestive tract diseases that do not permit them to absorb food nutrients, calcium supplements may be necessary. If a woman has undersized parathyroid glands, she may also need extra calcium. It is the enlargement of the parathyroid glands during normal pregnancy that allows the increased calcium absorption.

Other vitamins

Greater quantities of vitamin A and several of the B vitamins may be necessary during pregnancy. The Food and Drug Administration's recommended daily allowances of vitamins for pregnant and nonpregnant individuals are reported in Table 1-2.

Vitamin A should not be used in excess because it is toxic in dosages of over 100,000 units daily. This is more than 10 times the dosage found in a typical prenatal vitamin pill, so there is little need for concern about them. Vitamin D is toxic when 50,000 units per day are exceeded, but prenatal vitamins normally contain no more than 400 units of vitamin D. Mineral oil taken as a laxative may prevent the absorption of vitamins A, D, and E, unless taken at bedtime.

Table 1-2 United States recommended daily nutritional allowances (USRDA)

Nutritional needs	Nonpregnant	Pregnant or lactating
Calories (kcal)	2100	2400
Protein (gm)	50	80
A (IU)*	5000	8000
D (IU)	400	400
E (IU)	30	30
C (mg)	60	60
Folic acid (mg)	0.4	0.8
Niacin (mg)	20	20
B_1 (mg)	1.5	1.7
B_2 (mg)	1.7	2.0
B_6 (mg)	2.0	2.5
B_{12} (mg)	0.006	0.008
Iron (mg)	18	30
Calcium (mg)	800 to 1200	1200

**IU*, International units.

Women who are strict vegetarians should be certain that they supplement their diets with vitamin B_{12}. Lack of this vitamin can lead to certain anemias and nervous system disorders in the mother.

Nausea during pregnancy

Nothing can spoil the excitement of pregnancy like "morning sickness," the nausea, vomiting, and indigestion that at least 50% of pregnant women experience during early pregnancy. It may be comforting to know that morning sickness may actually be a good sign, indicating that hormone levels are rising as they should. Morning sickness, which can occur at any time of day, will usually not last longer than the first 3 months of pregnancy. If it does, consult your doctor.

Dietary adjustments should be the first method of controlling morning sickness. Obstetricians now recommend alternating dry foods and liquids in small quantities a couple of hours apart. The old standby, soda crackers, can be part of this regimen, but more nutritious foods, particularly protein, should be included too. Upset stomachs will tolerate chicken, fish, and mild cheeses better than some of the heavier red meats, beans, or nuts.

Bananas are an easily digested, nourishing food. Citrus fruits, tomatoes, and other highly acidic foods will probably not stay down. Cooked green vegetables rather than raw ones may be preferable during bouts of morning sickness.

Bendectin*

For the most stubborn cases of morning sickness obstetricians often prescribe the antiemetic (anti-nausea and vomiting) drug Bendectin. Bendectin is composed of pyridoxine, which is vitamin B_6, and doxylamine succinate, an antihistamine. Many women feel reluctant to use this controversial drug because it has been accused of causing birth defects. A well-publicized lawsuit was launched in 1980, charging that Bendectin was responsible for the birth defects of a child born in 1975. The judge finally decided that the case was ambiguous, and nothing was awarded the family. Nevertheless, the unfavorable effects of the publicity have caused the sales of Bendectin to drop off considerably. This, combined with the costs of legal defense, has probably been responsible for the substantial rise in the price of Bendectin. A 30-day supply now costs almost $60, whereas a few years ago it cost only $5 to $7.

Subsequent research has failed to show conclusively that there is any connection between Bendectin and birth defects. The Food and Drug Administration claims that Bendectin, the most studied drug under its jurisdiction, should be taken only if truly necessary, even though it has never been proven to cause a birth defect.

We believe that Bendectin is as safe a drug as any that will be found on the market today. Several studies, the most recent concerning more than 2000 women and babies, have shown that the drug has caused no ill effects. If nausea from pregnancy cannot be tolerated or controlled with dietary adjustments, we recommend its use. Because it is so important to eat correctly, it may be appropriate for your physician to prescribe it, if it is necessary to take the drug to be able to eat.

---

*NOTE: The Merrell-Dow Pharmaceutical Company decided to cease production of Bendectin in June 1983 because of adverse publicity based on unscientific evidence. The therapeutic gap caused by the loss of this widely used drug should prompt us to reflect on the effects litigation is having on the health care community.

Other drugs to control nausea

A category of drugs known as the phenothiazines (promethazine [Phenergan], prochlorperazine [Compazine]) can also be used in resistant cases of nausea, but these drugs are not approved by the FDA during pregnancy, although no birth defects have been shown to be associated with their use. They may be familiar to you because they are commonly prescribed to control motion sickness.

Common side effects of antinausea drugs include drowsiness and relaxation. Using analgesics (pain killers), sedatives, and alcohol along with these drugs is not advisable because the combination may create even further sleepiness. Driving or any other actions that require coordination are unwise when you are taking the antinausea drugs either alone or with other substances.

Once again, these drugs must be kept away from children. If a child has swallowed Bendectin or Compazine, always call for help. The child should be made to vomit, using syrup of ipecac as directed, and then be given activated charcoal to absorb the poisonous material. Vomiting should be induced very carefully because there is a chance that the child will lose motor control and breathe the vomited material into the lungs. In both instances a fast trip to the Emergency Room is indicated.

A new drug delivery system pioneered by the ALZA Corporation for absorption of drugs through the skin has been recently introduced. The drug is called Trans Derm I and is a small plastic patch that is applied behind the ear to control motion sickness. It contains a drug called scopolamine, which has been used for many years during labor with no known deleterious effects on the fetus. It may show promise for controlling nausea and vomiting in pregnancy.

Antacids

Heartburn, indigestion, and gas are frequent consequences of pregnancy, especially in the last few months as the baby grows larger and the mother's internal space is more crowded. Avoiding spicy and acidic foods and eating small frequent meals will help with the problems of heartburn and indigestion. Many physicians recommend sleeping with the head, neck, and shoulders slightly elevated to the right side to prevent acid from coming back up the esophagus (food tube). Bland foods like crackers near bedtime may also assist in controlling the symptoms.

Antacids do not seem like medicine, and there may be a temptation to swallow some every time a little discomfort occurs. However, they should be reserved for cases of severe heartburn or indigestion and after dietary adjustments have proved unsuccessful. We recommend antacid liquids such as Gelusil, Maalox, Riopan, Digel, Kolantyl, or Phillip's Milk of Magnesia, rather than chewable tablets. These may be purchased at any drugstore over the counter. Rolaids, Alka-Seltzer, and Bromo-Seltzer contain sodium, and pregnant women should probably avoid using them.

Personal experience

Barbara G, 26, worked part time as a secretary and cared for her husband and 3-year-old boy at home. When she was pregnant with her son, she had felt extremely well and had virtually no discomforts or medical problems. With her second pregnancy she had considerably more demands on her time and energy and soon began to notice that she did not feel as well. Almost immediately she had frequent bouts of nausea and indigestion. Her morning cup of coffee and her afternoon chocolate bar were replaced by saltines, soup, and toast. She refused to take Bendectin and began to control her nausea and vomiting with frequent small meals, alternating between dry and wet foods. Her doctors persuaded her not to use Alka-Seltzer or Bromo-Seltzer, which she had been in the habit of taking for heartburn prior to her pregnancy.

Barbara's morning sickness went away after her fourth month, but she found herself coping with nose colds and sinus infections throughout the windy and damp winter of her second trimester. Her doctor reminded her that she needed plenty of fresh fruits and vegetables in her diet. She took Sudafed as a decongestant and an occasional dose of Tylenol to relieve general discomforts and headaches. In her eighth month her entire family came down with a violent gastrointestinal flu. Barbara was very ill, and her doctor thought she might become so dehydrated she would need to be hospitalized. She took Kaopectate to relieve her diarrhea and stayed in bed for more than a week. Her appetite gradually came back, and she drank as many liquids as she could manage to get down. She eventually recovered, but she was concerned that the health problems she had had throughout pregnancy would adversely affect her baby.

Her doctor told her that the baby would gain a large proportion of its weight during her last month, as much as 3 pounds. He emphasized the need for Barbara to eat especially well at this time and told her to be particularly conscientious about getting enough protein.

Two weeks after her recovery from the flu, after a short but intense labor, Barbara gave birth to an apparently healthy girl weighing 7 pounds 3 ounces. She requested sterilization after the delivery, declaring that her child-bearing days were over as far as she was concerned. Because of her relatively young age, her doctors counseled her to reconsider this decision, and after some thought she decided to use a low-dosage estrogen birth control pill as a contraceptive method.

THINGS TO REMEMBER

1. Proper diet is a highly important part of pregnancy, and it is the one aspect over which a woman has the most personal control.
2. The most important dietary supplement is iron, and every pregnant woman should take it by the start of her fourth month of pregnancy.
3. Other vitamins may be helpful, particularly if a woman has an inadequate diet. Vitamins should never, however, be regarded as a substitute for nutritious food.
4. Nausea in the first 3 months of pregnancy is quite common and should disappear by the beginning of the fifth month. Dietary adjustments should be tried first, but if they do not work, Bendectin can be prescribed.
5. Occasionally, if nausea and diarrhea are persistent and dehydration occurs, a woman may need to be hospitalized and fed intravenously to restore normal body balance. She should not attempt to "put up with" truly disabling nausea, but should tell her physician immediately so that the necessary steps to provide relief can be taken.

2 Drug Effects on the Unborn Baby

The thalidomide babies of the 1960s were a particularly graphic and painful example of possible drug effects on the fetus. Images of the unfortunate children, armless and legless, have remained with us even after 20 years. It would probably be fair to say that this series of incidents formed public opinion about drug use during pregnancy more than any other situation in recent memory. The revelation in the 1970s that the widespread use of diethylstilbestrol (DES) to prevent miscarriage resulted in cancers and genital tract disorders in young women added fuel to the fire. Today many women believe that no drug can be safely taken during pregnancy. Women will suffer for months with nausea, endure respiratory and urinary tract infections, and refuse even a cup of tea or coffee for fear of damaging their unborn child. Our purpose in this chapter is to reassure prospective mothers that there is a middle ground out there, and that they do not necessarily have to endure illness or discomfort to protect their babies from harm. On the other hand, indiscriminate use of drugs is definitely out of place during pregnancy. Women need to be aware of the large variety of substances that fall under the category of drugs, what their own drug consumption habits are, and what they must do to minimize drug use while remaining healthy and happy expectant mothers.

How drugs affect the fetus

To understand the effects of drugs on the fetus growing in the womb, it is necessary to know something about the interrelationship between the mother's body, the placenta, and the fetus. Studies of pregnant animals have disclosed that drug concentrations in the umbilical cord and blood of the newborn correlate closely with the levels in the blood of the mother. In other words, if a mother takes a drug, it will end up in the fetus in nearly the same amounts that exist in her own bloodstream, especially if she has been taking the drug for an extended length of time. The placenta is like a big sponge, sucking up as many of the substances in the mother's bloodstream as it can. What she swallows, both good and bad, eventually gets to the baby. The placenta, with its many receptor areas where exchange of substances takes place, is quite large and would equal a rug laid out in a room 16 feet by 16 feet if it were flattened out to one layer.

Some drugs can reach the fetus in a matter of minutes: ampicillin, penicillin G, cephalothin, kanamycin, tetracycline, streptomycin, diazepam (Valium), phenytoin (Dilantin), phenobarbital, alcohol, aspirin, and propranolol (Inderal), a popular heart medication. A few substances will attain higher levels in the fetus's bloodstream than in the mother's—Valium being a prime example. Therefore it is especially important to avoid these drugs or use them only if absolutely necessary. The dosage received is definitely a factor in determining the impact of a particular drug. Because its organ systems are not fully developed, a fetus excretes and metabolizes (breaks down) drugs more slowly than does an adult, and this is another way the concentrations can build up, even if they have not initially entered in high dosages. The total exposure of the fetus to a drug over the long range is probably more important than a single high dose of drug at any given time.

How a drug will affect a fetus partially depends on the age of the fetus at the time it is exposed to the drug. Exposure to a teratogenic agent (one that causes defects) in the first 5 weeks following the last menstrual period sometimes results in miscarriage. During the fifth through the twelfth weeks after the last period major organs are formed, and a teratogenic drug may have an effect on their development. Beyond 12 weeks, delay in the unborn baby's growth and brain development is a major concern. Most defects are difficult if not impossible to diagnose before the baby is born.

The interplay between two or more drugs (drug interaction) may also pose a hazard to the fetus. For instance, drug *A* may be dangerous only in the presence or absence of drug *B*. Adding drug *C* may create an entirely new situation.

After birth the newborn remains susceptible to drugs that have crossed the placenta during labor and may exhibit their effects for hours or even days. The newborn's kidneys and liver are still not mature enough to excrete or metabolize drugs efficiently, so this may delay the exit of drugs from the newborn's system even further. Almost any drug circulating within the mother can be transferred into the breast milk or colostrum and thus reach the baby through that route. Generally speaking, however, we want to encourage mothers to continue breast-feeding, even if they must take a drug for a while when nursing. Newborns do not necessarily absorb the drugs acquired in breast milk through their immature gastrointestinal tract, and for the most part the benefits of breast-feeding outweigh the drawbacks of the drug transfer. If there is a question, always seek your doctor's advice.

Drug-taking habits of pregnant women

Studies show that women do take drugs during pregnancy; in fact, the average woman consumes two or three different drugs while pregnant. Excluding vitamin and iron preparations, 82% of all pregnant women take a prescription drug while they are expecting their babies, and 65% take drugs that have not been prescribed by a physician. Caffeine, alcohol, tobacco, and vitamins are used so routinely that sometimes people lose sight of the fact that they too are drugs. A study of several hundred pregnant women showed that marijuana, diet pills, and birth control pills were the three drugs most commonly taken at the time of conception. For women overall, pregnant or nonpregnant, tranquilizers and other mood-altering drugs are among the most commonly prescribed substances. The most commonly prescribed drug today is diazepam (Valium), a tranquilizer.

Two facts can be stated: (1) drugs taken by a mother-to-be definitely do get to the fetus; (2) the majority of pregnant women take drugs, both prescribed and nonprescribed. For these reasons the expectant mother should have up-to-date knowledge on which drugs can be taken with relative safety, and she, with the advice of her physician, can decide the benefits of a given drug versus its hazards.

A small number of drugs are clearly harmful to the unborn

baby, and these account for no more than 5% of all recorded birth defects. Hereditary and environmental factors cause another 30%, and for the remaining 65% the cause remains unknown. Several drugs have aroused suspicion, and we recommend caution in their use. An even larger number of drugs have at one time or another been associated with a particular disease. In this latter category the evidence is too sparse for us to make specific recommendations. The tables in this chapter give a detailed list of such drugs, with the findings to date, and readers, along with their physicians, can evaluate them for their own purposes.

All drugs should be used with caution during pregnancy. This includes over-the-counter drugs and habitual drugs like alcohol, tobacco, and caffeine. Drugs should be taken only for a specific reason and in the lowest possible dosage, for the shortest amount of time needed to get results. Pregnant women should let their doctors know of any drugs they are taking or are likely to take, including those purchased over the counter.

Drugs with known harmful effects on the fetus

At this point in time the number of drugs definitely known to produce a specific birth defect are few. They are listed, along with the problems they create, in Table 2-1. If at all possible, use of these drugs should be avoided during pregnancy, except phenytoin (Dilantin), used for treating epilepsy. In women with serious medical conditions like epilepsy, blood clots, or cancer, the use of teratogenic agents must be carefully considered along with the seriousness of the mother's need for the drug. The final decision lies with the woman and her doctor.

The DES story

In the early 1950s and 1960s a sizable number of women received diethylstilbestrol (DES), a form of high-dose estrogen, to prevent threatened miscarriage. About 15 years later a small number of girls who were born to these women were found to have diseases of the reproductive tract. Our two principal concerns when we examine these "DES daughters" is whether they have cellular changes in the upper vagina or cervix or structural deformities of the uterus and cervix.

Cells not normally found on the vaginal surface may be glandlike and resemble cells normally found on the inner lining of the

Table 2-1 Drugs known to cause birth defects

Drug	Birth defect
Anticonvulsants Trimethadione Phenytoin	Facial dysmorphogenesis (characteristic facial expression), mild mental retardation, growth retardation
Anticoagulants Coumadin and congeners	Nasal hypoplasia (underdeveloped nose bridge), stippling of bones, optic atrophy
Alcohol	Fetal alcohol syndrome: growth retardation, mild mental retardation, increase in anomalies
Folic acid antagonists Methotrexate Aminopterin	Abortion, multiple malformations
Hormones	
Diethylstilbestrol and congeners	Vaginal adenosis, carcinogenesis, uterine anomalies, epididymal anomalies
Androgens	Masculinization of female fetus
Methyl mercury	Central nervous system damage, growth retardation
Thalidomide	Phocomelia (short limbs)

cervix. This finding, known as adenosis, is very common among women exposed to DES during their mothers' first 3 months of pregnancy, but it does not cause any symptoms. The extent of the cellular abnormality can be determined in the doctor's office by inspection of the upper part of the vagina and cervix using special, washable stains. Because of the different chemical changes that take place in the vagina, once in a great while these abnormal cells undergo further changes, which are cancerous. This serious disease is known as adenocarcinoma. Fortunately, these changes occur only once in about every 10,000 women who have adenosis. We tell this to our DES-exposed patients to reassure them, and we do not treat their adenosis, other than to have the women come in annually for a pelvic examination and Pap smear. In those rare cases of adenocarcinoma, surgery and radiation treatment are usually very successful, especially if the cancer is detected early.

A second, and perhaps more worrisome, condition is the DES-exposed woman who is pregnant or has had repeated miscarriages. Certain defects tend to occur in the female reproductive organs of DES-exposed women that make it difficult to carry through with a pregnancy. They and their locations are listed below:

1. Upper vagina: vaginal septum
2. Cervix: cervical hood, cockscomb cervix, incompetent cervix
3. Uterus: T-shaped uterus
4. Fallopian tubes: distortion as the tube enters the uterus

Even though these defects are more commonly found in DES-exposed women, they are not common, and we seldom see them in the women we examine.

Many women come to us greatly concerned because they are uncertain about whether they were exposed to DES. We do not take any sort of action for these women until they reach their childbearing years. If, after a pelvic examination, there is no evidence of adenosis or abnormalities, we offer reassurance that they are unlikely to have problems. If a woman has an abnormal Pap smear or if staining of the vaginal cells suggests adenosis, we will continue to watch her and certainly treat her if that is necessary. If she has any of the deformities just listed or if she has had several miscarriages or premature deliveries, we will perform an x-ray examination of her reproductive tract (the x-ray technique known as the hysterosalpingogram). Under most circumstances we cannot correct these deformities surgically, but at least we can be aware of the deformities and watch very closely for signs of miscarriage or premature delivery during pregnancy.

Drugs with suspected harmful effects

Other drugs, again not a large group, have raised enough suspicion that doctors recommend that their patients avoid these substances during pregnancy. Table 2-2 lists drugs that we strongly suspect cause harm to the fetus and the effects that they can have. When more extensive and detailed studies have been completed, these drugs may move up into the proven-to-be-harmful category. Right now, we recommend that these drugs be avoided if at all possible, but we do not recommend that you automatically terminate a pregnancy because you have been using them. Chances are still in your favor that your baby will not have a birth defect or other problem. It might be possible to find a safer substitute, as in the case of the sulfonylureas for treatment of diabetes, or a woman can consciously choose to discontinue use of the drug, as in the case of nicotine.

Table 2-2 Drugs suspected of causing birth defects

Drug	Suspected birth defect
Alkylating agents	Abortion, anomalies
Hormones Oral contraceptives Progestins	Limb and heart defects
Lithium carbonate	Ebstein's anomaly (heart defect)
Nicotine	Growth retardation
Sulfonylureas	Anomalies(?)
Tranquilizers Benzodiazepines	Facial clefts

Drugs without proven adverse effects

This category is a rather sweeping one, for it covers the majority of drugs on the market today. Some of them have been studied in animals, and adverse effects were noted somewhere along the way. Yet results of research in animals clearly do not always apply to humans, and what may harm an animal may do nothing whatsoever to a human. The converse is also true. Thalidomide was studied extensively in animals, and no harmful effect was ever noted. What researchers could not know was that only in humans was a particular by-product of thalidomide formed, and it was this by-product that caused the malformations. Single reports of birth defects that could be associated with drug-taking abound in the medical literature, but the evidence is too scanty for physicians to draw definite conclusions. We can say at this time that, if a pregnant woman needs to take these drugs, they will do no obvious harm to her unborn baby as far as we know.

A long list of apparently safe drugs and their reported effects in human infants appears in Table 2-3. Only the generic (chemical) names of the drugs are listed. Often several manufacturers will market the same drug under different trade names.

Drugs most commonly used during pregnancy

Eleven of the drugs most commonly used during pregnancy are discussed, along with our recommendation for their use.

Table 2-3 Reported effects from drug exposure on the human fetus

Drugs	First trimester effects	Second and third trimester effects
Analgesics		
Acetaminophen	None known	Kidney toxicity
Narcotics	None known	Depression, withdrawal
Salicylates	Frequent reports, none proven	Prolonged pregnancy and labor, hemorrhage
Anesthetics		
General	Anomalies, abortion	Depression
Local	None known	Slow heart rate, seizures
Anorexics		
Amphetamines	Possible heart defects	Irritable, poor feeding
Phenmetrazine	Possible skeletal anomalies	None known
Meclazine	Facial cleft(?)	None known
Antiinfection agents		
Aminoglycosides	Possible nerve and kidney anomalies	Kidney and hearing toxicity
Cephalosporins	None known	Positive neonatal cultures
Chloramphenicol	None known	"Gray baby" syndrome(?)
Clindamycin	None known	Unknown
Erythromycin	None known	None known
Ethambutol	None known	None known
Ethionamide	Anomalies	None known
Isonazid	None known	None known
Metronidazole	Mutagenesis(?)	None known
Nitrofurantoin	None known	Anemia
Penicillins	None known	Positive neonatal cultures
Rifampin	None known	None known
Sulfonamides	None known	Anemia, low platelet count, jaundice
Tetracyclines	Impaired bone growth	Impaired bone growth, stained deciduous teeth (enamel hypoplasia)
Trimethaprim	None known (theoretical concern)	Jaundice
Anticoagulants		
Coumadin	Underdeveloped nose, eye abnormalities, stippling of bones	Bleeding, stillbirth
Heparin	None known	Bleeding, stillbirth
Anticonvulsants		
Barbiturates	None known	Bleeding, withdrawal
Carbamazepine	Unknown	Bleeding, withdrawal
Clonazepam	None known	Withdrawal, depression
Ethosuximide	None known	None known
Phenytoin*	Intrauterine growth retardation, craniofacial abnormalities, mental retardation, hypoplasia of fingers	Hemorrhage, depletion of vitamin K-dependent clotting factors

Continued.

Modified from Iams, J.D., and Rayburn, W.F.: Drug effects on the fetus. In Rayburn, W.F., and Zuspan, F.P., editors: Drug therapy in obstetrics and gynecology, Norwalk, Conn., 1982, Appleton-Century-Crofts.

*Proven teratogen.

Table 2-3 Reported effects from drug exposure on the human fetus—cont'd

Drugs	First trimester effects	Second and third trimester effects
Anticonvulsants—cont'd		
Primidone	None known	Hemorrhage, depletion of vitamin K-dependent clotting factors
Trimethadione*	Mental retardation, facial disfigurement	Hemorrhage, depletion of vitamin K-dependent clotting factors
Cancer chemotherapy		
Alkylating agents	Abortion, anomalies	Underdeveloped gonads, growth delay
Antimetabolites		
Folic acid analogs (metho trexate)*	Abortion, intrauterine growth retardation, skull anomalies	Same as above
Pyrimidine analogs (arabinoside)	Same as above	Same as above
Purine analogs (cytosine, 5-FU)	Same as above	Same as above
Antibiotics (actinomycin)	Same as above	Same as above
Vinca alkaloids	Same as above	Same as above
Cardiovascular drugs		
Antihypertensives		
Methyldopa	None known	Anemia, bowel contraction
Guanethidine	None known	
Hydralazine	Skeletal defects(?)	Fast heart rate
Propranolol	None known	Slow heart rate, low blood sugar, intrauterine growth retardation with chronic use
Reserpine	None known	Lethargy
β-Sympathomimetics	None known	Fast heart rate
Digitalis	None known	Slow heart rate
Cold and cough preparations		
Antihistamines	None known	None known
Cough suppressants	None known	None known
Decongestants	None known	None known
Expectorants	Fetal goiter	None known
Dextromethorphan	None known	None known
Diuretics		
Furosemide	None known	Death from sudden decreased blood flow to the fetus

*Proven teratogen.

Table 2-3 Reported effects from drug exposure on the human fetus—cont'd

Drugs	First trimester effects	Second and third trimester effects
Diuretics—cont'd		
Thiazides	None known	Low platelet count, low potassium, low sodium, jaundice
Fertility drug		
Clomiphene	Genetic abnormalities(?)	Unknown
Hormones		
Androgens*	Masculinization of female fetus	Adrenal gland suppression(?)
Corticosteroids	Cleft lip and palate in animals, not in humans	Growth delay
Estrogens	Heart anomalies	None known
Progestins	Limb and heart anomalies, VACTERL syndrome	None known
Hypoglycemics		
Insulin	Does not cross placenta	None known
Sulfonylureas	Anomalies(?)	Suppressed insulin secretion (unstable blood sugar levels)
Laxatives		
Bisacodyl	None known	None known
Docusate	None known	None known
Mineral oil	Decreased maternal vitamin absorption	Decreased maternal vitamin absorption
Milk of magnesia	None known	None known
Psychoactive drugs		
Antidepressants, tricyclics	Limb defects(?)	None known
Benzodiazepines	Cleft lip or palate(?)	Depression, floppy infant
Hydroxyzine	None known	None known
Meprobamate	Heart anomalies(?)	None known
Phenothiazines	None known	None known
Sedatives	None known	Depression
Thalidomide*	Phocomelia in 20% of cases	None known
Lithium	Facial clefts; Ebstein's anomaly (heart defect)	None known
Thyroid drugs		
Antithyroid	Goiter	Goiter (large thyroid), airway obstruction, hypothyroid, mental retardation
^{131}I*	Abortion, anomalies	
Propylthiouracil	Goiter	Same as above
Methimazole	Aplasia cutis (bald spot), goiter (large thyroid)	Same, aplasia cutis (bald spot)
Thyroid USP	Does not cross	None known
Thyroxine	Does not cross	None known
Tocolytics		
Alcohol*	Fetal alcohol syndrome	Intoxication, floppy, lethal

Continued.

Table 2-3 Reported effects from drug exposure on the human fetus—cont'd

Drugs	First trimester effects	Second and third trimester effects
Tocolytics—cont'd		
Magnesium sulfate	None known	Hypermagnesemia, respiratory depression
β-Sympathomimetics	None known	Rapid heart rate, cool body temperature, low calcium, inadequate blood sugar control
Vaginal preparations		
Antifungal agents	None known	None known
Podophyllin	Mutagenesis(?)	Laryngeal polyps(?), central nervous system effects(?)
Vitamins (high dose)		
A	Urinary tract and genital tract anomalies(?)	None known
B	None known	None known
C	None known	Scurvy after delivery
D	Mental retardation, facial cleft	None known
E	None known	None known
K	None known	Hemorrhage, if deficiency
Antiasthmatics		
Theophylline	None known	Decreased respiratory distress
Terbutaline	None known	Rapid heart rate, cool body temperature, low calcium, inadequate blood sugar control
"Street" drugs		
LSD	None known	Withdrawal
Marijuana	None known	None known
Methaqualone	None known	Withdrawal
Heroin	None known	Respiratory depression, withdrawal
Methadone	None known	Withdrawal
Pentazocine	None known	Withdrawal
Cocaine	None known	Withdrawal
Other		
Cimetidine	None known	None known
Caffeine	Anomalies(?) in high doses	Jitteriness
Azathioprine	Skeletal defect(?)	None known
Nonoxynol 9	None known	None known

*Proven teratogen.

Aspirin and acetaminophen

Aspirin and acetaminophen (Tylenol, Datril), when used in moderation, have not caused problems that we know of in the early stages of fetal development. There is some evidence that prolonged aspirin use in the last 3 months of pregnancy causes bleeding problems, prolonged onset and duration of labor, and premature closure of a major heart-lung artery in the fetus before birth. We recommend that aspirin be avoided in the last third of a pregnancy and that acetaminophen be substituted if a pain-killing remedy is needed. Heavy doses of acetaminophen must be avoided, however. Acetaminophen is often recommended as a substitute for aspirin, but more time is needed to study it before definitive conclusions can be drawn about its safety. Acetaminophen is toxic to the liver if taken in very large doses.

Decongestants

Pregnant women often suffer from nasal congestion and upper airway infections, which can last for the full 9 months. Studies have shown that decongestants containing pseudoephedrine (Sudafed) are not implicated in birth defects. Brompheniramine, chlorpheniramine, and meclizine, which are antihistamines with decongestant effects, have been studied in pregnant women, and no increase in birth defects was noted. They also appear to be relatively safe when used during nursing. Despite these favorable reports, we recommend that they be used in the lowest possible dosages. Whether nasal spray is a safer alternative to oral decongestants is unknown.

Antacids

Heartburn and indigestion will often plague a woman during pregnancy and intensify in the later stages because of increased pressure on the abdominal organs. Antacids are safe when taken in normal dosages, but several factors need to be kept in mind. Some antacids, such as Alka-Seltzer, Rolaids, and Bromo-Seltzer, contain sodium (salt). Pregnant women with salt limitations should read the labels carefully and avoid antacids with high sodium content. Antacids can cause constipation, which is also a common side effect of pregnancy, and they can cause decreased or delayed absorption of nutrients and certain drugs. A woman should discuss the use of antacids with her doctor if she is taking them in combination with any other drug, particularly antibiotics. We believe the liquid antacids such as Gelusil, Maalox, Mylanta, and Riopan are more effective than the chewable tablets, although the tablets have the advantage of being easy to carry, so you can have them with you at all times.

Penicillins

The two most common infections encountered during pregnancy are urinary tract infections and upper respiratory tract infections. The penicillins are commonly used to treat respiratory problems, and ampicillin is sometimes used for urinary tract infections.

Many studies have shown that penicillin does not have any adverse effect on the developing fetus, and in most of its forms it should be safe for pregnant women who are not allergic to it. On the other hand, the penicillins will appear in breast milk and may cause diarrhea and candidiasis, a type of oral fungus infection, in the nursing infant with long-term exposure. These drugs may have more adverse effects in later pregnancy, when the fetus absorbs drugs more efficiently. Penicillin is found in a variety of different forms, the more common of which are ampicillin, amoxicillin, penicillin G, benzathine penicillin, methicillin, nafcillin, carbenicillin, dicloxacillin, and ticarcillin.

Marijuana

We strongly discourage marijuana smoking during pregnancy. The active ingredients, carbon monoxide and tetrahydrocannabinol, cross the placenta easily and may depress the fetus's central nervous system. Charges that marijuana causes chromosomal damage are still largely unproved, and no specific pattern of birth defects has emerged. The major hazards appear to be similar to those of cigarette smoking—reduction of oxygen to the fetus and admission of potentially toxic materials through the placental membrane.

Antiemetics

Antiemetics are drugs that help reduce the discomforts of nausea and vomiting, which can be very intense during the first few months of pregnancy. The most commonly used antiemetic drug is Bendectin, which contains pyridoxine, a form of vitamin B_6, and doxylamine, an antihistamine. No adverse effects have been proved, and we recommend Bendectin if nausea and vomiting cannot be controlled by eating small, frequent, dry meals, alternating with liquids. (See Chapter 1 for further commentary on Bendectin.)

Promethazine (Phenergan) and prochlorperazine (Compazine) are also used for morning sickness; although they appear to be safe, they can have unwanted side effects such as drowsiness, disorientation, low blood pressure, and difficulty in walking or sitting properly. Unlike Bendectin, these two drugs have not been approved by the U.S. Food and Drug Administration for use during pregnancy.

Diet pills

Many women take diet pills before they know they are pregnant, and perhaps even as a result of the weight gain and fluid retention, which can begin very early for some expectant mothers. These pills sometimes contain amphetamines, powerful stimulants that affect the central nervous system. Studies have not shown any clear relationship between the use of amphetamines and birth defects, but the drugs are still suspect by many physicians. Other substances commonly used in diet pills, such as phenylpropanolamine, caffeine, and methylcellulose, have not been proved to be teratogenic. Diet pills should, however, be immediately discontinued once pregnancy is discovered because of the need for good nutrition at that time.

Caffeine

Caffeine is found not only in coffee, but also in tea, chocolate, cola drinks, headache tablets, diet pills, and cold and allergy capsules. It crosses the placental barrier without difficulty and has been detected in the blood and urine of newborns. It also appears in breast milk, and even moderate doses can produce jitteriness and irritability in infants.

In September 1980 the Food and Drug Administration suggested that pregnant women limit their consumption of caffeine severely, primarily as a precautionary measure. Since then almost 15,000 pregnant women have been studied by researchers at both Harvard and Boston universities, and no link between caffeine consumption and birth defects in humans has been found. Currently, we believe that caffeine is a relatively safe drug to use during pregnancy, but we still recommend that its use be kept to a minimum. Certainly, pregnant women should consume no more than 600 mg of caffeine per day, the equivalent of about 4 cups of coffee.

Birth control pills

Obviously, once a woman discovers she is pregnant, she will want to discontinue the use of birth control pills. There can be a period, though, when she continues to use them because she does not realize she is pregnant. Some problems have been associated with the use of birth control pills during early pregnancy. One of these is a defect involving the spine, anus (rectal opening), esophagus (food pipe), trachea (windpipe), and the arms and legs. It is known as the VACTERL syndrome. According to some reports, undersized limbs and heart defects are associated with birth control pills use early in pregnancy. Women should be reassured that the overall incidence of these defects is apparently no more than 3% among those who have taken contraceptives while pregnant. The odds are still overwhelmingly in their favor that they will bear a normal child if the pregnancy is continued.

Tobacco

Four thousand separate compounds have been identified in cigarette smoke, but the two most studied are nicotine and carbon monoxide. There is no longer any doubt that smoking can have a negative effect on an unborn infant. Low birth weight, problems with the placenta that result in hemorrhage, premature rupture of the membranes surrounding the fetus, and newborn death all have been documented. Nicotine causes changes in the mother's circulation and heart rate and seems to lower the baby's oxygen consumption. It can appear in noticeable amounts in the breast milk of heavy smokers. Carbon monoxide, a highly dangerous substance (famous for killing people who sit in garages with their car engines running or turn on their gas stoves without lighting the oven), also crosses the placental barrier easily. It competes with oxygen for a place in the blood of the fetus and can lead to insufficient weight gain and retarded growth. More studies need to be done on the effects of smoking in terms of actual birth defects, miscarriage, and slower mental function, but physicians already know enough to strongly recommend that their pregnant patients stop smoking altogether.

Alcohol

For decades doctors have suspected that alcohol usage was involved in some birth defects, and in 1973 a landmark study described a group of associated abnormalities that came to be known as *fetal alcohol syndrome.* These include nervous system disorders, growth deficiencies, and facial abnormalities. Mental retardation is also common. Undersized heads (microcephaly), the so-called water heads (hydrocephaly), and incomplete development of the brain occur.

What does it take to produce these results? Recent studies indicate that a daily intake of six or more "hard" drinks (whiskey, vodka, gin) or an equivalent of 12 bottles of beer or 12 glasses of wine significantly increases the chances of these abnormalities developing in the fetus. The effects of light or moderate drinking are not as clear cut. No absolutely safe level of consumption has been determined, so all pregnant women are cautioned to reduce alcohol drinking to the barest minimum, or to none at all, and to concentrate on eating well.

Personal experience

Tami T was 17 and a senior in high school. Her mother took her to the doctor immediately when she suspected that the plump teenager might be pregnant. Her fears were confirmed when the doctor announced that the pregnancy test was positive, and he estimated Tami to be about 14 weeks along. Tami took the news in stride, although she seemed uncertain about her plans for marriage or just how she would take care of the baby. Her mother was very upset, feeling that caring for her other three children and unemployed husband was all she could possibly handle. She was also deeply concerned about a number of substances Tami had been using at the time she became pregnant. Tami smoked both cigarettes and marijuana, and her boyfriend had been using cocaine for the past 2 years. Like so many of her friends, Tami used Dietac from time to time to try to lose weight, and she had been taking the drug for the past 4 weeks. The doctor's interview revealed that Tami had taken birth control pills sporadically. Frightened when she missed her period, Tami had gone back on the pill, even though she was already pregnant.

Tami's mother did not believe in abortion, but she was very fearful that if Tami did have a baby it might be defective because of all the drugs she had been using. Tami's doctor referred her to the high-risk pregnancy clinic at the state university medical center 65 miles away. In a conference with one of the obstetricians there, Tami and her mother were told that they would not advise an abortion purely on the basis of Tami's drug history. The risk of birth defects from any one of the drugs involved was less than 5%. The doctor did qualify her remarks by stating that she did not know if the particular combination of drugs might be more dangerous for the unborn infant's development.

After many discussions and arguments Tami's mother resigned herself that her 17-year-old daughter was going to have a baby. Tami is now 6 months pregnant. She has refrained from smoking and all other drug use. Her diet consists of too much junk food, but she takes her prenatal vitamins regularly. A community agency offers childbirth preparation classes for teenage mothers, and she is able to attend some high school courses so that she may graduate before the baby arrives. She and her boyfriend are still undecided about marrying.

THINGS TO REMEMBER

1. The important things to remember about drugs and pregnancy are that the unborn baby will be affected not only by the type of drug, but by:
   - **a.** The amount of drug actually reaching the fetus.
   - **b.** The individual genetic differences of both the mother and the child.
   - **c.** The age of the fetus at the time it is exposed.
   - **d.** The length of time over which a fetus is exposed to the drug.
   - **e.** The presence and interaction of two or more drugs.
2. We do not advise the use of either amniocentesis or ultrasound to test for drug effects on the fetus in most cases, since the results are not satisfactory for proving or disproving the effects of drugs.
3. Only a few drugs definitely or probably cause birth defects (pp. 21-24). Those should be avoided unless the medical benefit to the mother outweighs the danger to the unborn child.

4. The effects of most drugs are not really known, although many appear to be safe.
5. Consult with your doctor before taking *any* drugs, even those which you used habitually before pregnancy or purchased over the counter.
6. If you have a definite medical problem and your physician has prescribed a drug, you should take it. Drugs that improve a mother's health will often benefit a fetus much more than they will harm it.
7. Do not feel you must have an abortion because you took a questionable drug before you knew you were pregnant. Discuss the problem with informed people and find out what the odds are of producing a defective infant.
8. Tell your doctor about any drugs used around the time of conception, in early pregnancy, or at present.

3 Medical Disorders and Pregnancy

Every woman thinks about her personal health during pregnancy. Although pregnancy is a normal physiological event and not a disease, it creates many profound changes and makes strong demands on the body. Nature has made it possible for most women to adjust to pregnancy with a minimum of problems. In fact, many women feel better during pregnancy than at any other time in their lives. A substantial number of women, however, go into pregnancy with an underlying health problem that adds stress and even danger to the situation. Sometimes these problems remain undiscovered until pregnancy; sometimes the mother is well aware of them in advance of conception. In either case very careful attention must be paid to the mother's underlying health problem and the treatment needed to control it.

About one in every five pregnant women has an underlying medical disorder. Great strides have been made in treating diseases that used to make completing a pregnancy impossible, and we are seeing a higher proportion of these patients all the time. The list of disorders that can complicate pregnancy is very long, but the seven most frequently seen ones are anemia, both iron and folic acid deficiency (Chapter 1); high blood pressure (hypertension); diabetes; thyroid disease, both overactive (hyperthyroid) and underactive (hypothyroid); epilepsy; phlebitis, that is, blood clots in the legs, pelvic region, or lungs; and obesity (overweight).

Besides her own well-being, the mother-to-be worries about the effect of her disease on her baby and the effect of the medication or therapy that must be used to control it. All the "big seven" just mentioned, except obesity, require the use of drugs in their medical management, and they are discussed in the following sections in more detail.

Hypertension

Hypertension is caused by constriction or tightening of the blood vessels of the body. To pump the blood through the body at the necessary rate, the pressure in the vessels must be higher than normal because their diameter is smaller. Some cases of hypertension are related to underlying heart disease or "hardening" of the arteries, but other cases seem to exist by themselves. Hypertension is often symptom free and for this reason is especially dangerous. People sometimes don't even realize they are hypertensive until it is too late and they suffer a stroke or other blood vessel damage.

There are four different types of hypertension found during pregnancy: (1) acute hypertension, also known as preeclampsia-eclampsia, pregnancy-induced hypertension, or toxemia; (2) chronic hypertension; (3) chronic hypertension with additional acute hypertension; and (4) transient hypertension, which occurs during labor or immediately after delivery and then subsides.

Acute hypertension

Acute hypertension means about the same thing as preeclampsia-eclampsia, toxemia of pregnancy, or pregnancy-induced hypertension. Pregnancy-induced hypertension is not completely preventable, but it is treatable. It is seen more commonly with first pregnancies and is a disorder doctors will watch for closely in first pregnancies. When it is discovered in the mild stage, its most dangerous complications can be avoided almost completely. If not treated in time, both mother and infant will suffer as a result of this disorder. The first symptoms are usually noticed after the twenty-fourth week of pregnancy and include swelling of the face and hands, blood pressure greater than 140/90 (or substantial increases over previous readings), and the presence of protein in the urine. One of the things the doctor looks for in the urine sample you leave at each visit is protein, which may indicate signs of preeclampsia.

Once the diagnosis of mild preeclampsia has been established, the pregnant woman will have to be hospitalized. She will be put on a regimen of complete bed rest and encouraged to lie on her side. Her only medication should be phenobarbital, 30 mg, three times a day, to relax her. She will need a nutritious diet. Within 3 days she should have a noticeable loss of water, and her other symptoms should begin to subside. If she is at term, the doctor may consider inducing labor.

With severe preeclampsia, blood pressure will rise even higher (to 160/100 or more), protein in the urine will increase, inadequate urination may occur, visual or mental disturbances arise, and there may be difficulty in breathing. A woman exhibiting these symptoms will need her blood pressure monitored frequently, and she should be given intravenous magnesium sulfate. This drug prevents convulsions, which sometimes result from preeclampsia. If a woman with severe preeclampsia has a convulsion, it is called eclampsia. We believe that, once the doctor has treated these symptoms adequately, labor should be induced and the baby delivered.

The important thing to remember about preeclampsia is that it is most common in first pregnancies (occurring in 8% of them). To prevent it, see your doctor early in pregnancy and at frequent intervals. Lie on your side in bed for at least 60 minutes per day, starting at 14 weeks of pregnancy, and maintain a nutritious diet high in protein.

Chronic hypertension

Chronic hypertension usually exists in the mother prior to pregnancy, whether or not she is aware of it. Pregnancy tends to provoke chronic hypertension, which is more common in women who have had two or more children. Even in its milder forms, it is dangerous to the fetus, and the fetal death rate ranges from 15% to 40% when the disease is left untreated.

The first course a physician takes with chronic hypertension after chest x-ray examination, electrocardiogram, and laboratory studies have been completed is to give the mother medication to control the hypertension. After 20 weeks any diuretic (fluid pill) being taken must be discontinued. If her blood pressure changes are not too great, the pregnant woman can monitor blood pressure herself at home at least twice a day, while seeing her doctor every week or two. It may even be possible to discontinue her high blood pressure medication, at least for a period of time. If her pressure continues to rise, hospitalization and bed rest will become necessary. The three most important things a woman with chronic hypertension can do for herself are monitor her blood pressure conscientiously, rest in bed on her side at least 2 hours per day, and eat a nutritious, high-protein diet.

Drugs used to treat hypertension

The challenge to the physician in treating hypertension is finding the right combination of therapy and drugs that will do a minimal amount of harm to the unborn child while adequately treating the mother.

Obstetricians prefer to avoid diuretics (fluid pills) during pregnancy because they suspect these drugs create undesirable side effects in both mother and child. The thiazide drugs are popular diuretics for nonpregnant women but have been associated with jaundice (a blood disorder), low sodium, and low platelet count (cells necessary for blood clotting) in the infant. Other diuretics, such as furosemide, ethacrynic acid, spironolactone, and chlorthalidone, have been studied less, and their use is recommended only in severe cases of water retention.

α-Methyldopa (Aldomet) is a substance widely used for blood pressure control. More studies of this antihypertensive medication have been made than of any other drug used for the same purpose. To date it appears to be safe for both mother and child, and it is the primary drug that we recommend for control of chronic hypertension in pregnancy.

Propranolol (Inderal) is also used extensively in the management of hypertension. At the present time we have insufficient information about its effects on the fetus to make strong declarations about its use. Some isolated reports have noted growth delay and slowed respiration and heart beat in newborns. If propranolol is unquestionably the appropriate drug to use in hypertension management, the lowest dosage should be taken.

Hydralazine (Apresoline) helps to dilate constricted blood vessels that cause symptoms of hypertension. Doctors have had a wide experience with it and thus far believe it is not harmful during pregnancy. Given in combination with methyldopa, it appears to be a relatively safe form of hypertension control. In cases of acute hypertension it will have to be given intravenously, although in less serious situations it is effective when taken orally.

The most important drug used in preventing the seizures that occur with severe preeclampsia and eclampsia of pregnancy is magnesium sulfate, usually given intravenously. The vast majority of obstetricians use this drug around delivery time when it becomes necessary to treat any worsening hypertensive complications. The drug does not actually lower blood pressure a great deal. Rather, it seems to prevent severe fluctuations in blood pressure, which are damaging to the fetus. Most studies have shown that it does not have severe toxic side effects for the mother and fetus when given in proper dosages. Excessive magnesium can cause a slowing down of muscular responses and ultimately breathing and heart rate for both mother and child. Calcium chloride counteracts the effects of excessive magnesium and can be given if symptoms are noticed.

Glandular disorders

Not too many years ago diabetic women whose pancreases did not produce enough insulin had little chance of carrying a pregnancy through to successful completion. The course of their pregnancies was riddled with dangers and complications for both mother and child. Women with disorders of the thyroid gland had numerous problems as well and often could not even conceive. With improved medical, obstetrical, and neonatal care remarkable progress has been made in treating these problems.

Diabetes mellitus

Diabetes is caused by a disturbance in one of the most important glands in the body—the pancreas—located just below and behind the stomach. When affected, the pancreas does not release insulin properly, and the body is unable to use the sugar in the blood for fuel. Diabetics typically feel hungry and thirsty all the time and experience weakness and great fatigue. Excessive sugar can be found in both their blood and their urine.

From 2% to 3% of women who become pregnant have some form of diabetes. Diabetic pregnancies are considered high risk because so many complications can arise from a deficiency of insulin. Mothers are subject to problems with their metabolism and blood vessels and sometimes to infections. Babies of diabetic mothers are susceptible to premature delivery, birth defects, metabolic problems, and breathing difficulties. However, with the advances that have been made in medical science, a diabetic mother under meticulous care today has a very good chance of bearing a living infant.

Like high blood pressure, diabetes is often unmasked by pregnancy. Pregnancy makes great demands on the metabolism, the system the body uses to heat and cool itself and to fuel itself for action. The hormones of pregnancy change the way sugar is used by the body for energy. These changes must take place so both the unborn child and the mother can receive the nutrition they need for health. In the second half of pregnancy insulin requirements are about twice those of nonpregnant women. The extra insulin available causes pregnant women to have lower blood sugar levels than they would normally because so much of their sugar and protein is being used by the placenta and ultimately the fetus.

In spite of these complex changes, most pregnant women tolerate the added demands on sugar and carbohydrate burning very well. Women with known or hidden diabetes will not be so fortunate. Their blood sugar levels will rise and continue to be high during their entire pregnancy; if left untreated, these high levels prove very dangerous to both the fetus and the mother. Therefore obstetricians must assist in controlling the blood sugar levels of pregnant diabetics very carefully through the use of insulin and diet.

In some cases a properly adjusted diet will do the trick. Caloric intake should be about 1800 to 2400 calories daily. About 45% of the calories should come from carbohydrates, 30% to 35% from fat, and 20% from protein. Twenty percent of the food needed is usually consumed at breakfast, 30% at lunch, 35% at dinner, and 15% as a late snack. Diabetic expectant mothers should avoid going for long periods without eating.

Oral drugs to control diabetes should not be used during pregnancy. Although helpful to the mother, they cross the placenta to stimulate the fetal pancreas. Subcutaneously injected insulin (insulin shots given just under the skin), on the other hand, will not cross the placenta and have no effect on the fetus. Most pregnant diabetics will have to have subcutaneous insulin, even those who have previously managed their problems with oral drugs or diet control. Since insulin must be taken every day, it is much more convenient if a woman can administer her own insulin. Many women need instruction on how to give themselves insulin injections, but we have never seen a woman who was not able to learn how to do this.

The length of time it takes for insulin to act and the duration it should stay in the bloodstream must be adjusted to each patient's individual needs. Improved, more purified insulin is being marketed today, and in the future it will be easier to take insulin in lower doses with fewer side effects. Usually the prospective mother's requirements for insulin will either decrease or remain unchanged during the first half of pregnancy, whereas they will almost certainly increase during the second half.

Diabetics also must be managed very carefully during labor and delivery. Blood sugar levels must be checked frequently so that neither too much nor too little sugar appears. Insulin may have to be administered every 4 hours and blood sugar levels adjusted with intravenous glucose injection. After delivery, insulin requirements will be lower than normal for several days, particularly if the mother is breast-feeding.

Insulin must be used very carefully because it can have side effects. The most dangerous of these is hypoglycemia, or too little sugar in the blood. Diabetics should always be prepared with a candy bar or other high-sugar food in their purses or pockets to counteract this problem. Allergic skin reactions may occur at the site where injections are administered but usually go away of their own accord. Fat just under the skin where the insulin is injected may begin to disappear. The site of injection should be changed regularly, and sometimes a more purified form of pork insulin will need to be used.

The pregnant woman's need for insulin can fluctuate widely during the course of her pregnancy, which is why she must visit her doctor frequently. The increasing demands of pregnancy, acute infection, drug consumption, and overactivity of certain glands may explain this greater need for insulin. Problems with the placenta, inactivity, kidney disease, inadequate food intake, or underactivity of certain glands may decrease insulin requirements. A diabetic mother-to-be must learn to become sensitive to the way insulin works in her body so that she can quickly and accurately report changes that require a dosage or even an insulin type change.

The care of diabetic pregnant women has been revolutionized during the past decade. We now ask the mother to participate actively in her care by following her diet carefully and doing home blood sugar determinations by pricking her finger with a device called an Autolet. Some women check their blood sugar four to six times a day, three times a week. This is the only way that tight control of blood sugar can be achieved with insulin.

Many fetal tests are also done to assess fetal health from the thirty-fourth week of pregnancy until the baby is delivered. Currently, we deliver infants of diabetic mothers at anywhere from 36 to 39 weeks so the babies do not gain too much weight, a common problem for diabetics. Around 65% of these mothers will require a cesarean section because their cervixes are simply too firm and closed for an induction of labor.

Thyroid disorders

The thyroid gland, located on the lower part of the front of the neck, is one of the master glands of the body. Its job is to regulate the metabolism of the body, which includes temperature, heart rate, and use of food calories. It is intimately connected with the function of several other important glands, such as the pancreas, the pituitary, and the adrenals.

During pregnancy the two most common thyroid disorders found are hyperthyroidism and hypothyroidism.

Hyperthyroidism. Hyperthyroidism means the thyroid gland overworks itself by producing too much of the thyroid hormone thyroxin. The swelling that often occurs in the neck with hyperthyroidism is known as goiter. Symptoms of an overactive thyroid are rapid heartbeat, weakness, increased appetite, shaking hands, and shortness of breath. Since these are often common complaints of pregnancy, an overactive thyroid gland may not be immediately detected during checkups.

Treatment of an overly active thyroid gland before pregnancy includes drug therapy, surgery, or radioactive iodine administration. During pregnancy drug therapy is the safest form of treatment and in fact is necessary to prevent serious maternal and fetal complications, such as thyrotoxicosis, a medical emergency. The two drugs recommended for treatment of an overactive thyroid are propylthiouracil (PTU) and methimazole (Tapazole). Under no circumstances should radioactive iodine be taken by pregnant women. It crosses the placenta readily and can have very damaging effects on the fetal thyroid, even in small doses taken for a short period of time. Propylthiouracil is preferable to methimazole in pregnancy because transfer through the placenta is thought to be less rapid. Propylthiouracil gradually lowers the amount of thyroxin stored in the body. The excess amounts are what cause the symptoms of hyperthyroidism. Anywhere from 3 to 6 weeks may be necessary for the full effect of the drug to be noticed. After satisfactory thyroid hormone levels are obtained, women may be able to discontinue their thyroid medications. Daily doses should not exceed 300 mg so that side effects to the fetus can be prevented.

Because it does transfer through the placenta, propylthiouracil may affect the fetal thyroid gland. An enlarged thyroid (goiter) has been reported in up to 10% of all infants who were exposed to thyroid medication prenatally. Fortunately, symptoms of a malfunctioning gland in newborns tend to disappear after a few days. From 70% to 95% of pregnancies in which thyroid medication is used have a favorable outcome with no lasting effects on the baby.

Propranolol (Inderal) can be taken to control the symptoms of an overactive thyroid, such as rapid heartbeat, shaking, and palpitations. As discussed previously, experience with its use in pregnant women has not yet been wide enough to declare its absolute safety. Up to this time, no significant disorders have been associated with its use.

Hypothyroidism. Hypothyroidism is much less common in pregnancy than is hyperthyroidism. Usually it occurs when a woman has been treated for an overactive thyroid by surgical removal of a large portion of her thyroid gland. Symptoms include tiring easily, intolerance to cold, slow reflexes, and general sluggishness. Once again, these overlap with many of the symptoms of pregnancy, and it may not be easy for a doctor to diagnose an underactive thyroid.

If a pregnant woman has this condition, she will have to take a thyroid hormone supplement. We recommend synthetic levothyroxine (Synthroid) because it is the drug that is best absorbed and best tolerated by pregnant women. Thyroid supplements do not pass the placental barrier in any great amounts and do not seem to affect the fetus. The only major complication with levothyroxine is overdosage, in which case the symptoms will be those of hyperthyroidism. The treatment is to check the levels of thyroid hormone in the mother's blood and adjust the dosage accordingly.

Epilepsy

Epilepsy is a set of symptoms caused by disturbances in the brain and other parts of the nervous system that produce an altered state of consciousness. This state may be represented by a vague feeling of withdrawal or being out of touch with the surroundings, by feelings of dread that something bad is going to happen, by depression, by odors or sounds or sights that aren't really there (hallucinations), and by complete unconsciousness. In its worst form epilepsy causes violent seizures, jerking, writhing, and stiffening of the body; there may even be moments when breathing comes to a temporary halt.

Epilepsy is one of the most common disorders in the world; it occurs in 0.5% of the entire world population, a number that runs into the millions. In most cases seizures start before the age of 18, so epilepsy is found widely in people of reproductive age. Advances in medicine have permitted epileptics to lead more normal lives, find partners, and bear children. Thus the likelihood of a woman with epilepsy becoming pregnant is quite high; epileptics represent between 0.33% and 0.5% of all pregnancies.

Because of social problems and medical hazards combined, epilepsy resulting in seizures must be treated, even during pregnancy. Seizures are not only bad for the mother, they are bad for the fetus because they can deprive it of oxygen and create high blood acid levels, a condition that is suspected to cause birth defects and perhaps brain damage. Unfortunately, some drugs used to control seizures have adverse effects on the fetus also. Minimizing their use while still maintaining effective seizure control is the main challenge for doctors managing pregnant epileptics. Because of the risks of using these drugs, a woman with epilepsy should carefully evaluate how important having a child is to her and what she is willing to cope with if the infant has problems.

Causes and types

Epilepsy has a wide range of causes, such as infections like meningitis or encephalitis, poisons like mercury, lead, or various drugs, birth trauma, and heredity. If a mother has the type of epilepsy without any known specific cause, the chances of her child developing it are about 2% to 3%, five times higher than the general population. It has many different forms, but most people have one of four major types: (1) grand mal epilepsy, (2) focal epilepsy, (3) psychomotor epilepsy, and (4) petit mal epilepsy.

Grand mal epilepsy is the most commonly recognized form of epilepsy, and it occurs either alone or in combination with petit mal or psychomotor epilepsy in more than 70% of epileptics. The violent seizures of epilepsy occur with the grand mal form. They are similar to the type of convulsion seen in eclampsia (also known as toxemia of pregnancy).

Focal epilepsy often begins with twitching of the thumb, big toe, or face and may limit itself to such a twitching episode. It can also go on to the same kind of convulsions found in grand mal epilepsy.

Psychomotor epilepsy is characterized by altered moods, disturbing thoughts, and visual distortions. The victim may also involuntarily smack her lips, chew, or make other motions. Other changes include salivation, perspiration, and dilation of the pupils.

Petit mal epilepsy is characterized by brief spells of absence from, or being out of touch with, the outside world. The victim may blink her eyes or roll them back, but frequently no one else even realizes that she has had a seizure. Petit mal epilepsy usually disappears after adolescence, so it is rarely seen in combination with pregnancy.

Treatment during pregnancy

At least half of all pregnant epileptics find that their seizures worsen during their pregnancies. This is probably due to some of the physical changes of pregnancy and because the levels of antiepilepsy (anticonvulsant) drugs in the blood become diluted as the mother's blood volume increases. More of the drugs become necessary to maintain seizure-controlling levels in the blood. Sometimes mothers discontinue the use of their anticonvulsants because they fear damage to their unborn child or because they are suffering from the nausea and vomiting of early pregnancy and simply can't keep pills down. We advise against this; the only situation in which we recommend discontinuing anticonvulsant medication is if a woman is planning to get pregnant and she has been seizure free for a long time.

Both epilepsy itself and its treatment have been found to have adverse effects on pregnancy. Some investigators have found a significant increase in complications such as vaginal bleeding, toxemia, prematurity, and low birth weight. Other areas of particular concern are birth defects, altered maternal use of folic acid (Chapter 1), vitamin D deficiency, and, in the newborn, clotting problems, depressed breathing and drug withdrawal. The death rate of infants born to epileptic mothers is twice that of the general population, although both are very low. One review of more than 2000 children of epileptic mothers who took anticonvulsants showed a larger than average proportion with cleft palates, skeletal defects, heart problems, central nervous system malformations, gastrointestinal defects, facial abnormalities, mental retardation, and problems with the genital and urinary tracts.

Nevertheless, most physicians feel that women with epilepsy must continue their medications while pregnant. The goal then becomes to control seizures while creating as few adverse effects on the fetus as possible. The following considerations should be kept in mind:

1. The drug used for controlling seizures should have the best possible balance between effectiveness and potential harm to the fetus.
2. Initially a single agent should be used in moderate dosages to see if seizures can be controlled.
3. If the levels of a single drug become toxic before they become effective, then a second drug should be added, with the dosages of both drugs kept to moderate levels.
4. If the second drug accomplishes complete seizure control, then the dosage of the first drug should be slowly decreased but not stopped.
5. Any changes in drugs should be made very slowly.
6. The levels of the drugs in the bloodstream should be checked frequently.
7. In some cases the woman and her doctor will have to accept the fact that seizures cannot be controlled absolutely.
8. Excessive weight gain and sudden fluid retention may increase the risk of seizures, and every attempt should be made to prevent them.
9. The most common reason anticonvulsants fail to control seizures is because the pregnant woman has not been taking an adequate dosage or the wrong drug or dosage is being used.

Drugs used for seizure control

For grand mal and focal motor epilepsy phenobarbital and phenytoin (Dilantin) are the first choices. Phenobarbital is probably less likely to affect the unborn child but may be more effective when used in conjunction with phenytoin. Primidone, carbamazepine, and valproic acid may also be used for the grand mal and focal motor forms of epilepsy.

Psychomotor epilepsy may be especially difficult to control, and primidone is the best agent to use. Phenytoin may be added, and phenobarbital, carbamazepine, and valproic acid are sometimes useful.

Although petit mal epilepsy is rare in pregnancy, if a woman is suffering from this form, her number one drug choice is ethosuximide, followed by acetazolamide or valproic acid.

Drug problems. Trimethadione (Tridione), which is used for petit mal seizures, has a high potential for producing birth defects and should not be used by pregnant women or even by women who might become pregnant.

Phenytoin (Dilantin) is taken by the majority of pregnant epileptics. Most physicians feel it has the potential to produce adverse effects on the fetus, including birth defects, blood clotting disorders, and mental retardation. The "Dilantin syndrome" is well known and consists of growth retardation, peculiar facial features, and mild mental retardation. The occurrence of these problems appears to be unrelated to the dosage of phenytoin received. Phenytoin does not appear to accumulate in very great levels in breast milk; thus breast feeding can be undertaken even if the mother is using this drug.

Phenobarbital is probably less harmful than phenytoin, but it also appears to have some undesirable effects, such as creating maternal folic acid deficiency and blood clotting disorders in the newborn infant. If a pregnant epileptic takes phenytoin, phenobarbital, or primidone, she will need extra folic acid throughout her pregnancy, and the newborn infant will need vitamin K. In addition, infants must often withdraw from it because it is an addictive drug and can cause respiratory depression and withdrawal symptoms at birth.

Blood clots

Blood clotting is one of the major medical problems seen during pregnancy. Thrombosis, thrombophlebitis, and embolus formation are all terms that refer to blood clot formation, primarily in the veins. When thrombosis occurs, a cluster of blood particles of different kinds becomes stuck together to form a clot, or thrombus. The danger with this is that the flow of blood through a vessel will be stopped, and important organs in the body might not receive enough blood. Thrombophlebitis is clot formation and inflammation that take place in a vein. An embolus is a clot that has moved from where it was first formed to a smaller vessel where it plugs the circulation. Deep vein thrombosis of the legs and feet, pelvic vein thrombosis or thrombophlebitis, and pulmonary embolus (clots in the lungs) account for 50% of the deaths and illnesses related to pregnancy.

Physicians think that the risk of clot formation during pregnancy is particularly high because venous blood flow is not as vigorous as in nonpregnant women, the blood is thicker and more prone to coagulate, and blood vessels are more susceptible to injury because of the added pressure put on them. In the last 3 months of pregnancy fibrin, one of the blood elements involved in clot formation, increases substantially. The postpartum period (time immediately after delivery) is also a time of the risk of clot formation.

Symptoms of clot formation include pain in the legs or feet, difficulty walking, swelling of the legs, feet, and ankles, and warmth or tenderness in a specific area. It should be mentioned that some of these are symptoms of varicose veins. These veins appear just under the skin. They do not have good valve action for returning blood to the heart and thus tend to swell and get lumpy. They are uncomfortable and at times unsightly but not dangerous unless associated with deep vein thrombosis.

Women with leg vein problems will benefit by wearing support hose, elevating their feet above the waist several times a day, and avoiding standing in one position for a long time. Walking is beneficial for varicose veins, however, because it stimulates circulation.

Women with a history of clotting disorders, anemic mothers, women with cancer, and women whose babies must be delivered surgically run a higher risk of forming blood clots. For these women we believe that some attempt should be made to prevent clot formation, particularly at the time of delivery. Minidose heparin given as injections just under the skin is the best anticoagulant (anticlotting) drug for pregnant women. It does not cross the placenta and thus has no effect on the fetus.

After delivery some women develop fevers. Most of these go away either spontaneously or with short-term antibiotic treatment. If the fever continues and no abscess or other type of infection is detected, the cause is probably pelvic thrombophlebitis. Full-dose heparin will be required to treat the problem. Full-dose heparin will also be needed in the treatment of any accompanying deep vein thrombosis of the legs and feet.

We do not recommend the use of anticoagulant pills during pregnancy. These oral anticoagulants cross the placenta easily. Coumarin and warfarin (Coumadin) both pose dangers to the unborn child, particularly during the early weeks of pregnancy when the baby's organs are forming. Hemorrhages are another danger when oral anticoagulants are used, especially behind the placenta, where a hemorrhage could affect fetal nutrition.

Obesity

Obesity (overweight) is not always regarded as a medical disorder, but in pregnancy we believe it is at least a potential one because of the number of complications associated with it. The clinical definition of obesity in pregnant women is anyone who weighs over 200 pounds. We generally consider anyone who is more than 20% over her recommended weight to be obese.

Obese pregnant women are more susceptible to high blood pressure, diabetes, and blood clots. Pregnancy is a time for these problems to show themselves, and that is why doctors routinely screen for them. Physicians will be even more cautious about observation and testing in obese women and will perform certain tests much earlier than in women with normal weights.

Delivery problems occur more frequently in obese women. They tend to have larger babies, which can prolong or complicate delivery. Cesarean sections are often necessary, usually more involved, and take longer. Obese women are more difficult both to anesthetize and to wake up. Tissue with a great deal of fat in it doesn't heal as well because it has poorer circulation, and the risk of infection is higher for the same reason. The need for blood transfusions is higher.

Nonetheless, we strongly advise against dieting during pregnancy or while trying to conceive, even if you are obese. You and your unborn baby need a nutritious diet, similar to that of any other pregnant woman. A gain of 20 to 25 pounds is acceptable, and dieting can be reserved for a time after the baby is safely delivered. Obese women often need nutritional counseling: even if they eat a lot, they may be eating the wrong foods. If you have been taking diet pills around the time of conception and early pregnancy, you should discontinue them until the pregnancy is over.

Personal experience

Meredith J, a plump young woman of 19, had not planned to become pregnant, but both she and her husband were happy when they got the news that they were to become parents. They were also worried. Meredith had had a serious problem with diabetes since she was 10, and she needed daily insulin injections along with a special low-sugar diet. During her first year in high school she had begun to have grand mal epileptic seizures and had to take Dilantin to control them. Her doctor was very forthright with her. He warned her that she had two diseases that were difficult to control during pregnancy and that there were risks to both Meredith and the baby. He also assured her that he would follow her pregnancy very carefully and that medical science had come a long way in the past 15 years in helping women with her problems.

Because she had heard that Dilantin was a hazardous drug for unborn babies, Meredith stopped taking it right after she learned she was pregnant. Two weeks later she had a grand mal seizure. She passed out, her arms and legs contracted violently, and she lost her breath for almost 2 minutes and began to turn blue. She was rushed to the hospital and admitted. The doctors immediately gave her oxygen, restrained her, and started her once again on Dilantin through an intravenous line. When she returned to her normal state of mind, the doctors urged her not to stop taking Dilantin again. They pointed out to her that depriving her fetus of oxygen during a seizure was even more life threatening than exposure to Dilantin. She reluctantly agreed to continue taking the drug.

For the rest of her pregnancy Meredith worked at the bank as a teller and maintained her normal activities. She was extremely careful about her diet, making sure that she ate four properly balanced meals a day. She took prenatal vitamins with extra folic acid to counteract the effects of Dilantin on her red blood cells. Because of the seriousness of her diabetes, she had to monitor her blood sugar four times each day using an Autolet system. Her insulin dosage increased gradually as her pregnancy progressed. Once a month she had blood drawn to test for the amount of Dilantin in her bloodstream. Twice the doctor had to increase the dosage of Dilantin she needed.

At the beginning of her ninth month Meredith began to have episodes of near unconsciousness, caused by her blood sugar dropping too low during the night. Her insulin was decreased and she was admitted to the hospital so the doctors could watch her closely. Because her baby appeared to be growing very large, as fetuses of diabetic mothers often do, the doctors decided to induce labor at the beginning of her thirty-eighth week. They ascertained that the fetus's lungs were mature enough to withstand early delivery and then administered oxytocin. She had an uncomplicated 8-hour labor and gave birth to a healthy 7-pound 10-ounce girl. She was thrilled that her infant was healthy, after her worrisome pregnancy, and both she and the baby did well post partum. After the delivery the doctors were able to decrease her insulin and Dilantin dosages.

■ Personal experience

Janis T, 32, discovered during her first pregnancy 2 years ago that she had pregnancy-induced high blood pressure. During that pregnancy she received Aldomet to control the hypertension but still had to have an early delivery because her blood pressure continued to rise as her pregnancy progressed. After her daughter was born, her blood pressure dropped and remained within normal range. She was not aware of any other symptoms such as headache or chest pain.

When she first visited the clinic during her second pregnancy, at the beginning of her third month, everything looked good. However, her blood pressure slowly began to rise as the weeks passed. Janis bought a home blood pressure kit to monitor her hypertension. At the beginning of her fifth month the doctors decided she ought to take Aldomet again, which kept her blood pressure down adequately until the beginning of her seventh month. At that point she was taking the maximum allowable dosage of 2 gm per day, but the results were not satisfactory.

Her doctor informed her that she would have to be hospitalized with complete bed rest to see if that, along with medication, would bring her blood pressure down. Janis at first objected because she actually felt well. After the doctor explained the dangers of high blood pressure on both her and the unborn baby, however, Janis agreed to whatever was necessary for their safety.

Janis had to lie on her left side, only getting up to use the bathroom. In addition to her Aldomet, she was given hydralazine. She asked if she could be given a fluid pill, like her brother took, or Inderal, which had been prescribed for her father, since both of them suffered from hypertension. Her doctors told her that they never prescribed fluid pills to pregnant women and that in their opinion not enough was known about Inderal to give it safely during pregnancy.

Janis was discharged after a week and spent 1 more month at home, resting on her side for several hours a day. With 4 weeks to go until her due date, Janis began to excrete protein in her urine, a strong sign that she was developing toxemia again. The doctors decided to perform a repeat cesarean, and Janis and her husband both concluded that it would be wise if she had her tubes tied. She was fortunate to become the mother of a lean but otherwise healthy 5-pound 4-ounce boy.

After delivery her blood pressure dropped and, with the continuation of Aldomet, remained in a normal range. She currently sees her internist several times a year to keep a close eye on her hypertension.

THINGS TO REMEMBER

1. Most of the time mothers will need to continue their medications during pregnancy. Women with medical disorders are often plagued by guilt because they must take drugs that might not be good for their unborn babies. The general health of the mother is very important to the health of the fetus, and the harm done by discontinuing needed medications may very well outweigh the benefits.
2. The intake of the medications must be controlled carefully under the watchful eye of a physician. No more than the minimum necessary dosages should be taken, and these should be taken for the shortest amount of time required for them to do their job.
3. Because the mother has about 2 extra liters of blood circulating during pregnancy, she will often need higher dosages of

her medication to get the same results she got when she was not pregnant.

4. A woman with a medical disorder should consult a doctor the moment she suspects she is pregnant. Until she has her first appointment, she should continue with her routine pattern of medication.
5. Ideally, the pregnancies of women with serious medical disorders should be anticipated so that medications which are safer for an unborn child can be started before conception takes place.
6. The pediatrician who is to care for the child should be made aware in advance of medications that the mother took during her pregnancy, so that if problems resulting from the medications occur, he or she can be prepared.
7. After delivery the need for dosages of medications may change. Therefore a woman must return to her regular physician so that she can resume her normal course of treatment.

4 The Pregnant Drug Abuser

The extent of drug addiction in pregnancy has probably been underestimated by both the general public and the medical community. Perhaps people are unaware of the problem, or perhaps they are unwilling to recognize the breadth and depth of this combined social and medical problem. Drug dependency during pregnancy involves all social classes and age groups. Not only does it encompass the heroin addict from an urban ghetto seen in a methadone maintenance program, but it also touches the middle class teenager who has been experimenting with a wide variety of street drugs and the overwrought mother of four children who has a Valium habit. More and more, physicians see cases of drug abuse among women from the affluent sectors of society. Withdrawal symptoms have been observed in babies whose mothers used such diverse substances as phenobarbital, alcohol, pentazocine (Talwin), propoxyphene (Darvon), nicotine, and caffeine.

Most people tend to think of drug abuse in terms of heroin or other narcotic-like drugs. Actually, the list of drugs to which a woman and her newborn can be habituated is quite long. A few of the well-known ones are marijuana, hashish, diazepam (Valium), pentazocine, chlordiazepoxide (Librium), cocaine, angel dust (PCP), phenobarbital, flurazepam (Dalmane), secobarbital (Seconal), amphetamines (Benzedrine, Methedrine, Dexedrine), methaqualone (Quaalude), and combinations of all these. Sometimes the prospective mother hides her habit so well that no one, including her physician, knows she is taking a drug until the baby is born and shows withdrawal symptoms. From a medical standpoint street drug use is nearly impossible to study, with the exception of heroin addicts who are followed in methadone clinics.

Diagnosis of pregnancy

Sometimes it is difficult to tell if a drug user is actually pregnant. Women addicted to a single drug or combination of drugs often have irregular periods and menstruation. Under more extreme conditions they may be ill from infections, malnutrition, and anemia, which produce symptoms similar to those of early pregnancy. Even pregnancy tests do not work very well with addicts because of the effects of the drugs on the test processes. In some cases only ultrasound testing, feeling movement, or actually hearing the fetus's heartbeat allows the user to know that she is going to be a mother.

Table 4-1 Effects of drug abuse on the mother and fetus

Drug group	Signs and symptoms of overdose	Withdrawal symptoms	Fetal effects
Alcohol	Unusual behavior, mostly depressant, with stupor, loss of memory, hypotension	Agitation, tremors	Small head, mental retardation, altered facial expressions
Cannabis Marijuana THC Hashish Hash oil	Pupils normal, eyes bloodshot; BP decreased on standing; heart rate increased; sensorium—clear, dreamy, fantasy; state, time, and space distorted	None	None known
Sedatives Barbiturates Chlordiazepoxide (Librium) Diazepam (Valium) Flurazepam (Dalmane) Glutethimide Meprobamate Methaqualone (Quaalude)	Pupils unchanged; BP decreased, ± shock; respiration depressed; tendon reflexes decreased; drowsiness, coma, lateral nystagmus, ataxia, slurred speech, delirium, convulsions	Tremulousness, insomnia, blink agitation, toxic psychosis	None

Modified from Zuspan, F.P., and Zuspan, K.J.: Drug addiction in pregnancy. In Rayburn, W.F., and Zuspan, F.P., editors: Drug therapy in obstetrics and gynecology, Norwalk, Conn., 1982, Appleton-Century-Crofts.

Risks to the mother and fetus

Many experiments have been performed with animals in an attempt to study the effects of drugs on the unborn. In spite of these, it is very hard to predict what will actually happen to human babies. Apparently the risk of genetic problems or obvious birth defects is no higher than in the general population, but we don't know if drug abuse has an adverse effect on brain development. For this reason and because drug abusers have many additional problems, we believe open and sympathetic abortion counseling should be offered to them early in pregnancy. Most will probably choose to continue their pregnancies and should be supported in doing so, but their abortion options should be clear to them.

Table 4-1 lists signs of overdose and characteristic with-

Table 4-1 Effects of drug abuse on the mother and fetus—cont'd

Drug group	Signs and symptoms of overdose	Withdrawal symptoms	Fetal effects
Stimulants Diet pills Amphetamines Cocaine Methylphenidate Phenmetrazine	Pupils dilated and reactive to light; respiration shallow; BP increased; tendon reflexes hyperactive; irregular heartbeat; dry mouth, tremors, hyperactivity	Muscle aches, abdominal pain, hunger, prolonged sleep, ± suicidal	Excess activity with increased kicks
Hallucinogens LSD Ketamine Mescaline Dimethyltryptamine Phencyclidine (PCP)	Pupils dilated; BP elevated; heart rate increased; tendon reflexes increased; face flushed; euphoria, anxiety, inappropriate affect, delusions, hallucinations, realization	No withdrawal symptoms	No known fetal effects
Narcotics Codeine Heroin Meperidine (Demerol) Morphine Opium	Pupils constricted; respiration depressed; BP decreased; reflexes hypoactive; sensorium obtunded	Flulike syndrome, agitation, dilated pupils, abdominal pain	Intrauterine withdrawal with increased fetal activity; newborn withdrawal

drawal symptoms for the most commonly abused drugs. The most typical signs of overdose for each group of drugs involve the woman's behavior and her blood pressure and pulse. Except for narcotics, central nervous system stimulants ("uppers"), or depressants ("downers"), symptoms are not always obvious as the drug is withdrawn. In cases of addiction to narcotics, barbiturates, or hypnotic drugs it is important to realize that the unborn baby is addicted to the same drug as its mother. Getting the newborn infant off the drug, known as detoxification, must be done carefully and gradually. Withdrawing from a drug can be a demanding physical experience, and for an unborn or newborn baby it can be overwhelming.

Because of methadone maintenance programs, we know more about controlling heroin addiction than addiction to other drugs. Methadone must be substituted for heroin and the drug levels decreased slowly. Too rapid a decrease could cause the baby to be stillborn. The baby must be monitored throughout the detoxification process. If the fetus's activity seems excessive, it may be a sign that the detoxification process must be slowed down. With drugs like phenobarbital or diazepam, gradual withdrawal using decreased dosages of the same substances may also be necessary.

Needs of the pregnant drug abuser

We make the following recommendations to the pregnant drug abuser:

1. Avoid physical and emotional stresses that cause you to take drugs (including alcohol) for relief.
2. Attend prenatal classes and groups designed specifically to help you work through issues related to drug use during pregnancy.
3. Use crisis intervention programs staffed by professionals and paraprofessionals (former drug addicts) to assist with marital and family conflicts during pregnancy.
4. Make sure your diet is balanced and nutritious; include recommended vitamin supplements containing iron and folic acid.
5. Go to childbirth preparation classes given either in your community or at the hospital where you plan to have your baby.

Physical problems

Among the medical complications created by drug abuse are anemia, bacteremia (bacteria in the blood), endocarditis (an infection in the heart, often found in people with defective heart valves), dental infections, retaining water in the tissues, hepatitis, phlebitis and poor veins, pneumonia, water in the lungs, septicemia (blood poisoning), tetanus (lockjaw), tuberculosis, bladder and urinary tract infections, and a wide variety of venereal diseases (VD). It may take several visits to the doctor's office before these problems are completely diagnosed and treated, so the drug abuser should be examined frequently even in the early months of her pregnancy.

Emotional problems and rehabilitation

When still under the influence of their drug habits, many women maintain an artificial sense of well-being and stay out of touch with their real problems and ways of coping with them. Once in a rehabilitation program, the pregnant addict is apt to come up against the fear, guilt, and shame she has previously masked with drugs. Sometimes she will simply revert back to her habit, unable to face the truths about herself that she has finally glimpsed. In other cases she will go "cold turkey," that is, abstain suddenly and completely from drugs, regardless of the discomfort it causes her. Both routes are usually undesirable in a pregnancy. Whether it is safe to go cold turkey depends on the drug, and a woman should seek help from a physician before she attempts to do it.

People with the urge to use addictive drugs can be quite manipulative; they may attempt almost anything to acquire the substances they want. Often they will substitute more easily acquired drugs for the ones they are trying to give up. Women who actually are using other drugs (particularly alcohol) concurrently with methadone comprise between 15% and 40% of pregnant addicts. When multiple drug abuse is involved in a pregnancy, fetal death rises as high as 30%, and the multiple drug user should be aware that she is taking this level of risk.

Nutrition

Once a drug addict's pregnancy is diagnosed, she must improve her nutritional status. Since many women abusing drugs also eat very poorly, their diets often need to be of even higher quality than in a normal pregnancy. If possible they should see nutrition counselors to help them achieve a diet that includes at least 100 gm of protein a day. Supplementary vitamins are also a must. At least 25% of drug addicts are anemic and will need iron supplementation twice a day plus additional folic acid.

Preparing for delivery

Remarkably, the incidence of delivery complications in drug-dependent women varies little from that of normal pregnant women. Premature rupture of the membranes (water bag) does occur more frequently, as much as 2⅛ times more often according to some studies. The babies themselves are often smaller than normal. The nursery team must be alert to the symptoms of withdrawal in the newborn. These include shaking, sweating, excessive yawning, unstable temperature, vomiting, diarrhea, rapid respiration, irritability, sleeplessnes, a shrill high-pitched cry, and seizures. After delivery the babies may need to receive the drug their mothers were taking in gradually decreasing amounts to help them withdraw with less discomfort.

■ Personal experience

Mandy L, divorced, jobless, and pregnant, was a street-drug abuser. Looking considerably older than her 23 years, the thin, stringy-haired blonde admitted to the obstetrician that she was taking PCP (angel dust), cocaine, and heroin when she conceived. Now about 4 months pregnant, she also confessed that she was still shooting heroin. She told her doctor that, in spite of her drug habits, she very much wanted her baby. The doctor reassured Mandy that she would do everything in her power to ensure a healthy infant; but she needed Mandy's commitment to cooperate with her recommendations. Nervously Mandy agreed to go on a decreasing methadone maintenance program.

Fortunately Mandy did not have gonorrhea, hepatitis, or any of the other infections often found among street-drug abusers. She was, however, anemic and badly nourished. Her doctor referred her to a government-funded community service agency, where a team of physicians, nurses, nutritionists, and social workers worked with her almost daily. With a government allotment she was able to purchase fresh fruit, vegetables, meat, milk, and prenatal vitamins. Even though she didn't keep her medical appointments regularly, Mandy managed to gain 30 pounds. Her anemia remained stable, neither improving nor worsening.

Mandy told her doctors she was willing to try to discontinue her use of heroin, but they informed her that, if she attempted to discontinue her drug habit, it could have harmful effects on her baby. She enrolled at the methadone clinic and started on a program where she received a daily dose of 80 mg of methadone. Her dosage gradually decreased until it was at 15 mg daily at the end of her pregnancy.

Because Mandy's periods had been irregular since she began using drugs, the date of her conception was uncertain. Her doctor used ultrasonic imaging to determine the age of her fetus, and she continued ultrasound testing throughout the pregnancy to check on the baby's development. Just about the time of the predicted due date, Mandy went into spontaneous labor and delivered what appeared to be a healthy 6-pound 5-ounce girl. The baby was watched carefully in the nursery for symptoms of drug withdrawal. She appeared to be slightly more wakeful and fussy than would be expected of a baby from a normal mother, but she ate well, and her irritability was decreasing at the time Mandy left the hospital with her.

Mandy was in reasonably good physical health at the time of her discharge. Her parents had decided to let her and the baby come back home with them. Mandy remained on methadone maintenance for 4 more months, and then the drug was stopped. She continued to see her social worker twice weekly and is now enrolled in vocational training classes at the local community college.

THINGS TO REMEMBER

1. Despite drug addiction, many women get pregnant and want to have their babies. They deserve the same support and assistance in completing a successful pregnancy as do any other pregnant women.
2. Apparently there is no obvious risk of birth defects or genetic damage associated with drug abuse in the mother. At this time we don't know what the effects on brain development are.
3. Diagnosis of early pregnancy in a drug abuser may not be easy. Because of the unknown risks to the unborn baby, the

option of abortion should be discussed in an open and sympathetic manner.

4. The extent of drug abuse or addiction at conception or throughout pregnancy is sometimes difficult to assess. The list of abused prescribed or street drugs is quite long, and the mother-to-be may hide her habit so well that she cannot receive adequate care.
5. The chances of an addict completing a successful pregnancy will be much higher if she is totally honest with her physician about the substances she is taking, and if she is willing to work at controlling her habit for the sake of the baby and herself.
6. Pregnant drug addicts often have many health problems. They need good medical attention, a highly nutritious diet, and supplemental prenatal vitamins containing iron and folic acid.
7. Not all pregnant women should go off their drugs "cold turkey." Depending on the drug and the doctor's impressions, they may need to go on a maintenance program with gradually decreasing amounts of the drug administered to them.
8. Pregnant drug abusers often need psychiatric attention, vocational counseling, and moral support, as well as good medical care. They may need help in turning their attention from substitute drugs such as alcohol.
9. Babies of addicted mothers may very well need a staged withdrawal program shortly after birth.

5 Pain Relief during Labor

In the past, women had to suffer pain during childbirth. Even after pain relief techniques had been developed, many cultural and religious beliefs prevented a woman from using drugs or techniques to obtain pain relief. Although nitrous oxide was discovered in 1772, it was not applied for the pain of childbirth until 75 years later. Women can thank Queen Victoria of England for her part in establishing the precedent of using drug relief for pain during labor. After she received chloroform during the birth of her eighth child, sanctions against relief of labor pain with drugs were lifted and the techniques of obstetrical analgesia (pain relief) and anesthesia began to develop.

Today a wide variety of methods are at the disposal of a woman about to give birth. They range from drugs that hypnotize, tranquilize, narcotize, and paralyze to techniques employing specific breathing patterns, autosuggestion, relaxation, and positive visualization. Acupuncture and acupressure massage have also become increasingly popular over the past few years. A woman can now custom design her own labor, employing different methods in the sequence she wants.

Our strong recommendation is that a woman do all she can to prepare for childbirth, in consultation with her doctor. Hospitals and private practices frequently offer preparatory courses, and many communities have adult education classes that teach Lamaze, LeBoyer, and Bradley methods, autogenic training, and other popular systems of giving birth. Probably as important as the particular techniques they teach is that these courses help to dispel fear, one of the greatest pain enhancers during childbirth. The mechanisms of childbirth are very powerful, and if a woman feels she has some control and knows what to anticipate, the enormity of it all diminishes to manageable size. A woman should be able to look forward to her delivery eagerly, knowing that she will experience one of the great achievements of her life. We strongly encourage women to become well informed about pregnancy, labor, delivery, and the subsequent care of their babies.

As with pregnancy, it is certainly better if a woman can go through labor and delivery without the use of drugs. However, between one third and two thirds of women giving birth will ask for and need some form of drug relief before the baby actually arrives. You should not feel guilty if you need some assistance. Enduring agony just so you won't have to use a drug is not helping you or your baby. Childbirth and labor go much more smoothly when the mother is as comfortable as possible under the circumstances.

If a woman wishes to use one of the nondrug techniques, she should also work out a contingency plan with her doctor that allows for drug relief if it is needed. Preplanning allows her to be involved in the choice of labor management and probably prevents the guilt and upset that some women feel when they find they must resort to drugs to help control pain. This is especially true for first babies, when the mother has few hints as to how her body is going to respond to the demands of labor.

The major reason for not using drugs during delivery is that they all have some negative effects on the baby. Another important consideration is the mother's wish to be totally aware of what goes on during delivery and to be alert and ready to welcome her baby. Mothers should know that contemporary drug management keeps them conscious most of the time and also that there are recommended drugs which have minimal side effects on the newborn. In other words, you can control pain effectively and still be awake when your vigorous, pink, crying baby is placed in your arms.

Systemic analgesia and sedation

Systemic medications are those which enter the bloodstream and are dispersed throughout the entire body, including of course the placenta and the fetus. Because the stomach and digestive system can be easily upset and absorption delayed during labor, these drugs will be injected or given intravenously, rather than as pills.

Narcotics

Narcotics are the most widely used systemic medications for reduction of pain during the first and second stages of labor. They have a profound effect on the central nervous system and work by modifying the impulses traveling to the pain centers there. The narcotic drugs commonly used during labor are meperidine (Demerol), morphine, alphaprodine (Nisentil), pentazocine (Talwin), and fentanyl (Sublimaze).

In mothers-to-be narcotics given in the small-to-moderate dosage appropriate for labor produce drowsiness, mental fuzziness, and pain relief, but not unconsciousness. They raise the pain threshold (level at which a person can tolerate pain) and reduce the feeling of pain. An advantage is that they do not affect the heart or blood pressure, an important consideration during labor. They may, however, induce nausea or even vomiting because they slow down gastrointestinal activity. Reports that narcotics speed up the process of labor have appeared, but this is probably because they greatly reduce tension and fear, not because of any effects they might have on uterine contractions.

The narcotics easily cross the placenta and can have a very strong effect on the central nervous system of the fetus. They may slow the baby's heart rate and breathing or cause alterations in the brain wave patterns. Meperidine, one of the recommended narcotics for labor, can cause respiratory depression in the baby if it is given 2 to 3 hours rather than 1 hour before delivery and if the dose is too large. Drugs such as naloxone (Narcan) may be given to the infant to reverse respiratory depression if it seems at all serious.

We believe that in most cases meperidine is still the best narcotic to use for pain relief during labor. If the mother has a great deal of nausea and vomiting, pentazocine may be preferable. Alphaprodine works very rapidly and for short periods of time and may be useful in certain situations. Fentanyl is a relatively new narcotic with very fast but brief narcotic action. It has not been widely used because any respiratory depression it causes in the mother or unborn infant outlasts its pain-killing effects.

Barbiturates

Barbiturates are sedative-hypnotics, that is, they relieve tension, slow the laboring woman down, and finally put her to sleep. Except for the early stages of labor, they are no longer widely used. The well-known barbiturates are thiopental (Pentothal), secobarbital (Seconal), pentobarbital (Nembutal), amobarbital (Amytal), and phenobarbital. In the relatively small doses of barbiturates that would be given during labor, adverse effects are rarely seen in the mother. They do not inhibit labor, cause only slight changes in heart action or blood pressure, and usually do not slow down breathing. The central nervous system is exquisitely sensitive to their effects, however, and even a small dose can depress it significantly, causing drowsiness and stupor. What is more, they cross the placenta very rapidly and take quick action on the fetus. If the expectant mother has used barbiturates excessively or if the doses given to her at labor are too high, the baby may have respiratory depression or exhibit abnormal nervous system reactions for the first 48 hours of life. He or she may not be alert and may have difficulty feeding. These problems are more likely to occur if the mother has received both narcotics and barbiturates during labor.

Tranquilizers

Tranquilizers have fallen out of favor for use during labor, except in mothers with specific medical disorders like epilepsy or eclampsia. Diazepam (Valium), chlordiazepoxide (Librium), and flurazepam (Dalmane) have all been used to relieve the mother's anxiety during labor. Diazepam, the most popular of the three, has also been especially helpful in controlling grand mal epileptic seizures and convulsions caused by eclampsia. The major objection to diazepam is that it crosses the placenta readily and can reach levels in the blood of the fetus that are higher than in the mother. It affects the fetal heart rate and in larger doses can cause limpness, poor feeding, and poor temperature control after delivery. The baby has great difficulty detoxifying this drug, and traces of it may be present up to 5 days after delivery.

Another group of tranquilizers, which are normally used for psychotic disorders like schizophrenia, can be employed during labor to control nausea and vomiting. These include promethazine (Phenergan), propiomazine (Largon), thioridazine (Mellaril), and perphenazine (Trilafon). They do not appear to affect the mother in any adverse way except to sedate her and make her indifferent to her surroundings. If they are used along with narcotics, the dosages of the narcotics may be lowered and the required effects still achieved. No detrimental effects on the fetus have been associated with these drugs, although placental transfer is rapid.

Inhalation agents

Gases that can be inhaled are occasionally used for pain relief during labor, even though their popularity in the United States has declined in recent years. They are still used frequently in the United Kingdom and Europe.

With close supervision the woman in labor can help herself by inhaling an agent when she feels a contraction coming on and stopping the inhalation as the contraction subsides. She must be able to remain conscious and cooperative, however. Usually three inhalations during the course of a contraction are adequate to control pain without putting the mother to sleep. Inhalation agents are also helpful when uterine relaxation must be obtained, such as when a second twin must be delivered, when the placenta must be removed by hand, or if the uterus needs to be repositioned.

Nitrous oxide is the best and safest agent to inhale for pain relief because it works fast and does not last long. As a side benefit, it provides extra oxygen to both the mother and the fetus. It is best when used during the late stages of labor. Methoxyflurane (Penthrane), halothane (Fluothane), enflurane (Ethrane), ether, and isoflurane have all been used for pain relief during labor but are not as safe as nitrous oxide. They may relax the uterus too much and promote bleeding. On the other hand, they are the best agents to use when uterine relaxation must be obtained.

The risks of inhalation agents during labor and delivery are several. In anesthetic doses, slowed maternal breathing may cause inadequate oxygen intake and loss of cough reflexes in the throat, which can result in accidental intake of the contents of the stomach into the windpipe. Antacids are usually given prior to the use of any inhalation anesthetic to cut down irritation of upper airways if anything is breathed in. All inhaled anesthetics cross the placental barrier and can briefly depress the fetus's brain, heart, and lung activity.

Amnesia drugs

Several years ago the amnesia drugs scopolamine and ketamine were in vogue. The idea was to put the mother in a dreamlike trance from which she would emerge unable to remember the "agonies" of labor. Nowadays women seem to prefer remembering their labor, and these drugs are seldom used. If the dosage is too high, they can cause hallucinations and delirium, which is another reason for avoiding their use. Scopolamine does not kill pain and so has to be used in combination with narcotics to produce the so-called twilight sleep.

Local anesthesia

Local anesthetics (Novocain-like drugs) are used to block pain in specific and limited areas without significantly affecting other parts of the body. Interestingly, local anesthetics are among the most widely used of all drugs during labor, and they have potentially some of the most toxic and long-lasting effects on infants and mothers. If a local anesthetic reaches the mother's circulatory system, her body systems may become depressed and she may even go into a coma. Such a problem might result when the local anesthetic is accidentally injected into a vein or artery. This hazard does exist in deliveries because the site of local anesthetic injections is usually rich in blood vessels, although it is very uncommon.

Local anesthetics should be prevented from reaching the fetus because it cannot metabolize these drugs as well as a baby or an adult, and thus the drugs stay "trapped" in their bodies for prolonged periods. In spite of potential problems, local anesthetics have been used relatively safely in obstetrics for a number of years. The problems should be minimal when the anesthesia is in the hands of a capable and experienced anesthetist.

The most typical use of a local anesthetic during pregnancy is when an episiotomy (a cut in the tissue surrounding the vaginal opening) is performed to prevent tearing of the tissues as the baby's head emerges. Episiotomies are performed in 85% of deliveries in the United States. Bupivacaine, lidocaine, mepivacaine, and procaine (Novocain) are all used for local anesthesia. We believe that bupivacaine (Marcaine) is the drug least likely to create undesirable side effects, and therefore we recommend it as the drug of choice for relief of local pain.

Regional anesthesia

Regional anesthesia, more popularly known as spinal anesthesia, is a form of local pain relief that has been popular for use during labor for several years. It is the most effective form of anesthesia because it offers satisfactory pain relief with few complications. A "spinal" can numb as much as two thirds of the body, from the breasts down (Fig. 5-1). Unfortunately, not all hospitals have anesthesiologists or obstetricians with the training and skills to give regional anesthesia, so it cannot be obtained everywhere. Two kinds of regional anesthesia are commonly used during labor and delivery: continuous lumbar epidural anesthesia and spinal saddle block anesthesia (Fig. 5-2).

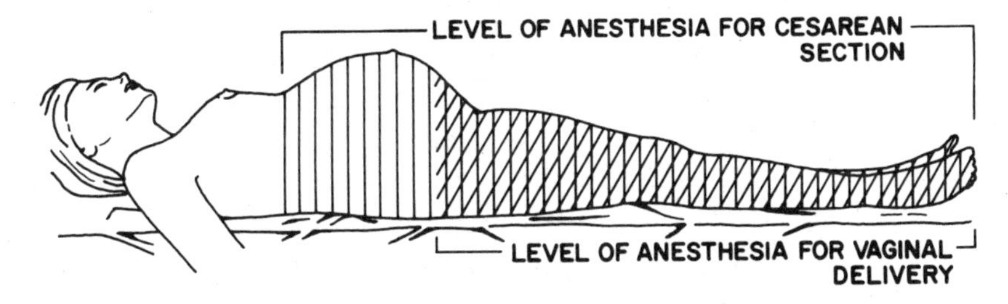

FIG. 5-1 Anesthetic levels for vaginal delivery and cesarean section. (Redrawn from Regional anesthesia in obstetrics [Clinical education aid no. 17], Columbus, Ohio, 1979, Ross Laboratories.)

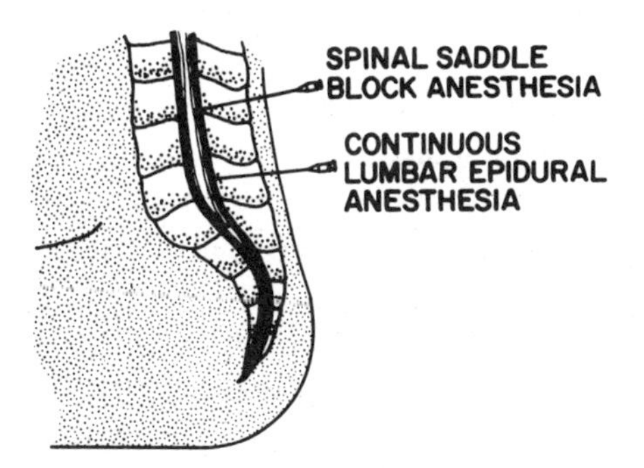

FIG. 5-2 Spinal saddle blocks and continuous lumbar epidural blocks are two kinds of regional anesthesia used during labor and delivery. (Redrawn from Regional anesthesia in obstetrics [Clinical education aid no. 17], Columbus, Ohio, 1979, Ross Laboratories.)

Epidural anesthesia

In some hospitals epidurals are used more commonly than spinal saddle blocks. They can provide pain relief for the duration of labor and may also be used for the anesthetic delivery, since the amount of pain-killing material injected will be regulated according to need. They are accomplished by placing a hollow needle into the epidural space (the outer layer of the spinal cord) where the nerves that travel from the spinal cord to the uterus and cervix lie. A tiny plastic tube is threaded through the hollow needle, which is then removed. The plastic tube is left taped to the mother's back until the baby has been delivered. Repeated doses of the anesthetic can be delivered through the plastic tube as needed.

The pain of contractions disappears within 10 to 15 minutes of the injection of a local anesthetic, usually bupivacaine or lidocaine. Once the anesthetic begins to work, the mother's feet and legs feel warm and heavy and tingle slightly, a pins-and-needles kind of sensation. Typically a dose of the drug administered will last at least 90 minutes, and then another injection will be needed. This form of pain relief is particularly helpful for women who have had long and difficult labors in the past, who are very fearful of labor, or who have great pain in early labor, with the labor expected to last a long time. Before an epidural block can be given, labor must be established with the cervix dilated at least 4 cm.

Epidural anesthesia is advantageous for women with high blood pressure who cannot tolerate other kinds of pain killers. In high-risk deliveries where the baby is in breech position, with twins, or with premature babies it is the ideal pain killer because it ensures that the mother's pelvic muscles are relaxed and the babies meet little resistance as they come out. Its major disadvantage is that the mother cannot sense the urge to push, even though she is capable of pushing, and forceps may have to be used to bring the baby through the birth canal. Both the mother's and the baby's progress has to be monitored more closely if epidural anesthesia is given. The mother will need an intravenous fluid infusion to keep her blood pressure from dropping suddenly, and the baby's heart rate must be monitored as well.

Epidural blocks are the preferred method of anesthesia for cesarean section deliveries in our medical centers. About 80% to 90% of mothers who must have a "c-section" receive epidural blocks; the rest undergo general anesthesia. With the epidural block the mother can be awake to see her child as it first emerges (without actually watching the operation), and it is a much more satisfying situation with the mother feeling like she has still taken part in the birth of her child. A stronger dose of anesthetic must be given for a cesarean section delivery, and the numbness must reach up the mother's body to just below the breasts.

Saddle block anesthesia

Spinal saddle block anesthesia is used toward the end of labor, often when it is apparent that a forceps delivery is necessary. A hollow needle is inserted deeper into the spinal cord until it reaches the spinal fluid, and the local anesthetic is then injected. The action of this method is very quick. However, it is a one-time only injection used for the end stages of delivery.

The drawbacks to spinal anesthesia are relatively few, but they should be mentioned. Sometimes the anesthetic does not completely numb the area it should, and localized pain is still felt. After a saddle block some women (less than 3%) have a headache of several hours' duration. This is caused by leakage of the spinal fluid and can only be cured by lying flat on the stomach until it goes away, usually when the small puncture wound heals up. To a certain extent spinal anesthesia will prolong labor, but with the mother in no pain and the infant closely monitored, this is usually not a problem. Because the baby doesn't descend into the birth canal as well when a spinal is used, up to 40% of babies have to be brought out with forceps. Many women regard this as a major disadvantage because of the potential for trauma to the baby's head and to the birth canal.

The idea of a needle going into the spine may be a bit frightening, and many women worry that they will become paralyzed or suffer some other type of injury to the spine. Provided that the anesthesiologist is skillful, the likelihood of this is remote; we regard spinal anesthesia as a very safe procedure, and we recommend it.

Finally, a mother's feeling that she will be missing something by not sensing the pain of contractions should not be underestimated. If a woman's need to be totally involved in the birth experience is high, then she will have to choose another method of handling pain.

Personal experience

Penny R, a 27-year-old nurse, had worked hard during her first pregnancy to prepare for her delivery. Both she and her husband attended Lamaze childbirth preparation classes, toured the hospital's labor and delivery areas, and discussed the birth process with her doctor. They strongly desired a natural childbirth, but their doctor convinced them to be open to other options as well. Eventually they developed a willingness to use whatever measures were necessary to ensure a safe and comfortable delivery.

Penny's water bag broke while she and her husband were sitting in front of the television set early on a spring evening. She was already 3 days beyond her due date, so she quickly gathered her things together and went to the hospital. By the time she arrived, her contractions were fairly strong and the delivery room doctor found that her baby's head was already engaged in her pelvis. He informed her that it should be only a matter of hours until she became a mother.

She walked around the labor hall for a short time but soon found that the intensity of the contractions was more than she could tolerate while on her feet. She reclined in a semisitting position on the narrow labor bed, and found that her Lamaze breathing techniques were more effective when she lay on her left side. Her husband gently massaged her lower back and the backs of her legs as he coached her through the increasingly intense contractions. The doctor recommended that she breathe a mixture of oxygen and nitrous oxide to make the contractions more tolerable. When her cervix had dilated to 6 cm, she found that she seemed to be losing control. The pain had become nearly unbearable, so she gave in reluctantly and asked for more pain relief. After determining that her infant was in a position that would likely require a longer labor than they had anticipated, the doctors gave Penny a dose of intravenous Demerol. Her pain was relieved somewhat, and she relaxed in a slightly dreamy but conscious state of mind. Ninety minutes later Penny gave birth to an 8-pound boy with a 5-minute Apgar score of 8. Although he seemed a little sleepy, no measures were taken to stimulate him, and within 24 hours his responses were perfectly normal.

Penny's cervix had been completely dilated for the last 90 minutes of labor, so the doctors performed an episiotomy, using

Xylocaine to numb the area of the incision. She bled heavily after her delivery because of a boggy uterus, and the doctors gave her Pitocin intravenously and massaged her uterus vigorously every 5 or 10 minutes. The bleeding cleared up within 30 minutes after delivery.

Although the childbirth process hadn't met Penny and her husband's expectations, they were pleased with the experience and not at all sorry that they had turned to additional pain relief measures when Penny needed them so badly.

THINGS TO REMEMBER

1. Childbirth preparation is very important. Methods of managing pain and other aspects of delivery should be discussed with your doctor, well in advance of delivery. Try to remain flexible and leave your options open.
2. Numerous drug-free methods of pain control are available, and it is a good idea to take classes if you are interested in natural childbirth. We recommend that everyone become well-informed about pregnancy, labor, childbirth, and care of the newborn.
3. One third to two thirds of women still need some drug relief during pregnancy, and even if you plan a natural childbirth, it is wise to think about what drugs you might need.
4. Low doses of narcotics like meperidine given intravenously seem to be most effective and least dangerous to the newborn.
5. Local anesthetics are used in 85% of women to control pain in the cervix, the external genitals, and the floor of the birth canal, particularly when an episiotomy incision must be made.
6. Regional anesthesia is a good method for women who want to block pain completely but still remain conscious. When a cesarean section is necessary, an epidural block is the procedure of choice for 80% to 90% of our women in labor.

6 Postpartum Care

After the mounting tension of 9 months of eager anticipation and the dramatic climax of a delivery, women often don't think about or prepare for the events of the immediate postpartum period. Nevertheless, this stage is as important in the whole cycle of pregnancy as any other. A mother must recuperate quickly and completely so she will have the strength and energy to care for her newborn infant. Both mother and infant need care immediately after birth to avert problems with potentially serious consequences.

Pain relief

The first thing a woman may notice after her attention wanders from her newborn infant is that she has some cramping pain caused by continuing uterine contractions. This is completely normal and, in fact, desirable because the uterus must work to expel whatever materials remain (to minimize further bleeding or any infection) and to return to its normal nonpregnant size, about that of a woman's fist. If she has had an episiotomy, she may feel discomfort at the incision site and find it hard to sit normally.

Typically, doctors prescribe aspirin or acetaminophen (Tylenol, Datril, Anacin III), or acetaminophen with codeine for these discomforts. As discussed in Chapter 10, prostaglandins appear to be the chief cause of uterine cramping. Not only do these drugs alleviate pain, but they also act as prostaglandin inhibitors. Sitz baths and topical soothing antiseptic pads are also available to help relieve episiotomy pain.

Uterine contracting drugs

Oxytocin

Shortly after delivery the obstetrical nurse or doctor massages the uterus vigorously and checks to make sure that it is indeed contracting. If it is flaccid or boggy, medication to make it contract is prescribed. Oxytocin (Pitocin, Syntocinon), a hormone produced in the pituitary gland, is the most widely used uterine stimulant. It causes uterine contractions both during labor and post partum and stimulates the release of milk from the breasts. Most obstetricians make sure that their patients routinely receive oxytocin after delivery.

Oxytocin should only be given intravenously when used for the induction of labor because its administration can be more easily controlled, and any sustained contractions are reversed by discontinuing the medicine. It may have serious side effects, and uterine contraction patterns must be watched carefully by the delivery room staff using internal or external monitoring devices. For effective use in stimulating postpartum contractions to prevent uterine hemorrhage, oxytocin is also usually given intravenously, and fewer hazards are associated with its use after delivery.

In all situations the need for oxytocin must be weighed carefully against its dangers. Prior to delivery it must be used cautiously when the mother is pregnant with twins, the baby is in breech position, the baby's head appears to be too large for the mother's pelvis, the mother has given birth many times before, the fetus is in distress, the mother has severe hypertension, there is excessive amniotic fluid, or the mother has had a prior cesarean section. We recommend that oxytocin not be used when a woman has had a repeat cesarean section with a vertical (up and down) uterine incision, the fetus is positioned on its side rather than coming head first, or the placenta is in front of the fetus at the cervical opening (placenta previa).

Side effects from oxytocin are infrequent when given post partum and usually occur only in women with previous cardiovascular (heart and blood vessel) problems. Cardiovascular side effects include premature ventricular contractions (early beats) and low blood pressure, usually when the oxytocin is given in combination with a general anesthetic, such as cyclopropane, or when infused rapidly.

Ergot preparations

The other drug in common use today to promote uterine contractions after delivery is ergot, a substance derived from the fungus *Claviceps purpurea.* Ergot has a much longer history than oxytocin, the first report of its usage being in 1582 in Europe. By the early 1800s it had been introduced into American obstetrical practice. Folk medicine suggests that ergot, when combined with quinine, can induce abortion. Along with oxytocin its effectiveness for abortion in early pregnancy is highly variable, and we do not recommend that it be used for this purpose.

The uterus is very sensitive to ergot stimulation, and powerful contractions may persist for hours. Ergot is therefore not appropriate for induction of labor, since it can damage the fetus by causing excessively strong contractions. It is best prescribed after delivery or following a miscarriage or abortion.

Ergonovine maleate (Ergotrate) and methylergonovine maleate (Methergine) are two ergot preparations that are taken by mouth or injected either intramuscularly or intravenously. Unlike oxytocin, ergot preparations are absorbed well in the gastrointestinal tract. The tablet form is usually taken three or four times per day for 3 days to 1 week to diminish uterine bleeding. Other than causing excessively strong contractions and cramping, ergot has few side effects. On uncommon occasions it will cause a temporary increase in blood pressure; so any mother with high blood pressure should not receive the medicine.

Ergot has been shown to be helpful in treating migraine headaches, but these preparations are not the same as Ergotrate or Methergine, and the latter should not be used for migraines.

Breast milk suppressants

Despite the increasing interest in breast-feeding today, many new mothers still choose not to breast-feed or cannot do so for medical reasons. It is certainly possible to meet an infant's nutritional needs with a good formula, and no woman should feel pressured to nurse her baby. Traditional methods of stopping lactation (the production of breast milk), such as breast binding, ice packs, and fluid restriction, have been replaced by the convenience of drugs that help to stop the flow of milk in a relatively comfortable fashion.

During the course of pregnancy the body prepares for the complex process of lactation: prolactin (the hormone for milk production), estrogen, and progesterone levels increase progressively. Breast tissue becomes firmer, and the breasts increase in size as pregnancy advances. A substance called colostrum may be discharged by the nipples prior to and shortly after delivery. It is yellowish white and is the precursor of breast milk.

Immediately after the baby is born, breast filling is triggered by hormones; after that, the major stimulus for continuing lactation is sucking by the baby or pumping of the breasts by mechanical means. When there is no sucking or pumping, the body reestablishes its normal hormone balance within a few days, and the milk in the breasts disappears gradually. Prior to this time, however, a significant number of women experience painful swelling and hardness of the breasts (engorgement) due to the milk coming in, and their breasts will leak, even if there is no pumping or sucking. For these women we recommend the use of one of the following drugs: bromocriptine mesylate, chlorotrianisene, or combined estradiol valerate and testosterone enanthate. The choice of drug depends on the route of delivery and duration of therapy.

Bromocriptine

Bromocriptine mesylate (Parlodel) is a nonhormonal agent that exerts its effects on the entire body rather than locally, as do other popular breast milk suppressants. Bromocriptine quickly abolishes the rise in prolactin levels and prevents the lactation process from continuing. This drug is taken by mouth twice a day for 14 days.

An advantage to bromocriptine is that it works in women whose breast milk has already been established, whereas the hormonal lactation suppressants do not have any effect in these women. Bromocriptine is also used to treat amenorrhea (lack of menstruation), premenstrual discomfort, galactorrhea (spontaneous milk production), and infertility caused by a failure to ovulate (Chapter 9).

Mild to moderate recurrence of milk production has been reported in up to 40% of women who discontinue bromocriptine use. The problem is usually handled by continuing the course of the drug for another 7 days. Uncommon side effects include headache, dizziness, and nausea. Bromocriptine is more expensive than the other lactation suppressants.

Chlorotrianisene

Chlorotrianisene (TACE) is a synthetic, estrogen-like drug that can be taken by mouth. Although not a hormone, it acts in a manner similar to that of estrogen by decreasing milk production. Taken orally, chlorotrianisene is stored in the fatty tissue of the body and released gradually where it acts specifically on the breasts. The recommended dosage is 1 capsule (72 mg) taken orally two times per day for 2 days, beginning within 8 hours of delivery. It may also be taken by mouth in dosages of 12 mg four times per day for 7 days or 24 mg four times per day, for a total of six doses. Chlorotrianisene appears to be an effective drug in about 90% of the women who use it. It apparently does not affect other postpartum changes in the body, such as lochial flow (blood and debris discharged from the uterus), return of the uterus to normal size, and return of menstruation.

Estradiol and testosterone

Deladumone OB and Ditate-DS are trade names for the compound composed of estradiol valerate and testosterone enanthate, both of which are hormones. Because there is a balance between the male (testosterone) and female (estrogen) hormones, the body does not suffer the ill effects it would if each were taken alone. This drug is given in a single 2 ml injection at the beginning of the second stage of labor or usually within an hour of delivery. Like chlorotrianisene, the drug acts primarily on breast tissue and does not affect other parts of the body. Studies have shown that less than 5% of the women taking estradiol and testosterone have symptoms of breast pain or engorgement. Because the drugs must be injected into the muscle, estradiol and testosterone treatment may cause swelling and pain at the site where the needle pierces the skin.

Rh factor and Rh immune globulin

One of the first prenatal tests made during pregnancy is identification of the mother's blood type. Everyone has red blood cells, but there our sameness ends. There are over 140 different kinds of proteins on the blood cell surface. These proteins are called antigens, and humans have a wide variation in the number and type of these proteins. If you have a particular antigen on your red blood cells, you are said to be positive for that antigen.

If you don't have it, you are said to be negative. One of the most important antigens is called the D or Rh antigen, more commonly known as the Rh factor. If the father of a child has an Rh-positive blood type and the mother is Rh negative, the infant is likely to inherit the father's blood type and be Rh positive. Genetic factors are significant in determining whether there is an incompatibility between the blood types of the mother and fetus. When the blood of an Rh-negative person is mixed with the blood of an Rh-positive person, antibodies are often made in the Rh-negative person to fend off or destroy the antigens of the Rh-positive red blood cells.

In an Rh-negative pregnant woman, if even a tiny bit of the unborn baby's blood reaches her bloodstream and it is Rh positive, she may produce antibodies. Although not harmful to the mother herself, these antibodies can cross the placenta and begin destroying the unborn baby's red cells. This phenomenon usually doesn't create problems during a first pregnancy because the blood of the mother and fetus rarely mix until late in pregnancy or at the time of delivery. Once antibodies directed toward Rh-positive blood cells are formed, they remain permanently in the mother's bloodstream and present a danger to any future fetuses. When the antibodies attach to the surface of the baby's red blood cells and weaken them, they produce a disease called hemolytic anemia, a potentially life-threatening condition for the fetus or newborn.

Fortunately, there is now a way around this potentially disastrous situation. The problem had been under investigation for several decades, and finally in the 1960s a method of preventing the antibody formation was developed. In 1968 a protein antibody called an immune globulin was developed and marketed under various trade names (Gamulin Rh, RhoGAM, MICRhoGAM, and HypRho-D). It is derived from women with Rh-negative blood who have formed antibodies from pregnancies and from Rh-negative men who have been deliberately immunized by repeated injections of Rh-positive blood and have formed antibodies from the red cell antigens.

Once injected into the muscle, the protein finds its way into the mother's bloodstream. When it encounters a red blood cell from the fetus, the antibody or immune globulin surrounds and coats the antigens on the cell surface. It thus prevents the mother's immune system from recognizing the cell as a foreign substance and forming antibodies [specifically directed against the $Rh_0(D)$ antigen antibodies]. Since widespread use began, the incidence of the destructive condition has declined from 4.5 to 1.4 cases out of every 1000 births.

The mother should be Rh negative and the infant Rh positive if the drug is to work. If the infant's blood type cannot be determined for some reason, then an injection should be given to an Rh-negative unsensitized mother anyway. The immune globulin should usually be given within 72 hours after delivery.

There is a slight risk of antibody formation before delivery, so many physicians advocate starting the Rh immune globulin program during pregnancy. A large study performed in Canada revealed that an injection given at 28 weeks' gestation and again at delivery prevented 98% of the women from forming antibodies. We routinely administer immune globulin to our Rh-negative unsensitized mothers between the seventh and eighth months, especially if the father is known to be Rh positive. Since the immune globulin will not remain in sufficiently high levels to prevent antibody formation at the end of pregnancy, an additional dose is needed at delivery.

Any Rh-negative woman undergoing an amniocentesis (withdrawal of amniotic fluid from the womb by needle) may need Rh immune globulin if she has a potential Rh factor incompatibility with her fetus. There is always a slight risk that the placenta will be pierced by the needle and a small amount of fetal red blood cells will cross into the mother's bloodstream, causing her to produce antibodies.

Even in early pregnancy about 2% or 3% of Rh-negative women who have a miscarriage or abortion will develop red cell antibodies. Before the twelfth week a small dose of immune globulin (MICRhoGAM) is necessary; after 12 weeks a full dose of Rh immune globulin should be administered (Table 6-1).

Immune globulin is a thick substance, and intramuscular injections must be given through a large needle. They may therefore sometimes cause pain, lumpiness, or swelling at the site of the injection. A short-lived fever may develop in a very few cases, and an allergic reaction to the foreign protein occurs rarely.

Major causes of failure of $Rh_0(D)$ immune globulin are (1) receiving it too late, (2) receiving an inadequate dose, (3) having the mother's Rh type misinterpreted, and (4) already having antibodies from a blood transfusion, previous pregnancy, or blood

Table 6-1 Indications and usual dosage of Rh immune globulin

Indications	Usual dosage
Gestational age less than 12 weeks	50 μg (microdose)
Abortion, spontaneous or induced	
Tubal pregnancy	
Threatened abortion	
Gestatational age more than 12 weeks	300 μg (minimum)
Abortion, spontaneous or induced	
Tubal pregnancy	
Amniocentesis	
Vaginal bleeding	
Premature labor (?)	
Delivery	300 μg (minimum)
Massive fetal-maternal hemorrhage	
Sterilization post partum or after abortion	

from the fetus entering the mother's circulation earlier in the current pregnancy. When antibodies have formed, under these circumstances this drug is not helpful.

Immediate newborn care

Perhaps 95% of all babies make the transition from life inside the womb to life outside without difficulty. Certain drugs, however, should be given to all infants. Regardless of their physical condition at birth, all babies need medication to prevent eye infections and possible bleeding. Some infants may require additional assistance in making this big adjustment.

Eye treatment

Doctors must administer a drug effective against gonorrhea organisms to the baby within an hour after delivery. The incidence of undiagnosed gonorrhea in certain pregnant women may be high, and estimates hold that 28% of babies born to mothers with gonorrhea will develop the infection in their eyes as they pass through the birth canal.

Silver nitrate has been used effectively for many years to prevent gonorrheal infection in the eyes of newborns. The single-dose ampule instilled into the baby's eyes right after birth exerts a direct germ-killing effect. Chemical conjunctivitis (a redness and irritation of the lids) occurs infrequently but may last for up to 1 week. Some argue that it temporarily impairs the baby's vision and interferes with the mother-infant eye contact that creates early bonding. We believe its value in preventing a damaging infection outweighs this factor and consider it a necessity in newborn care.

Tetracycline and erythromycin eye ointments, both antibiotic preparations, have also been shown to be effective against gonorrhea. In addition, each drug destroys *Chlamydia trachomatis,* a microorganism that also causes newborn conjunctivitis and respiratory tract infections. Except for reports of local mild irritation and rarely an allergic reaction, neither ointment produces apparent side effects. They are significantly more expensive than silver nitrate, which probably explains the much more common usage of silver nitrate.

An injection of penicillin G used to be given to newborn infants within the first 30 minutes of life to prevent gonorrhea. We do not recommend this form of treatment, since the gonorrhea organism has undergone a number of mutations (change in structure) over recent years and often resists treatment by penicillin. Furthermore, many people develop a local irritation and a few a dangerous allergic sensitivity to penicillin, and blood tests have demonstrated the potential for this problem in babies who receive a single intravenous dose of penicillin G.

Bleeding problems

The newborn baby, especially if born prematurely, has only 20% to 40% of an adult's ability to clot blood. Vitamin K assists greatly in the formation of blood clotting factors. It is therefore necessary to give vitamin K (AquaMEPHYTON) until the infant's body adapts to food intake and begins to form its own vitamin K. Babies who do not receive vitamin K run the risk of hemorrhage in the gastrointestinal tract, umbilical cord, circumcision site, nose, or other areas inside the head within the first 48 hours of life. Breast-fed newborns are also susceptible to this problem because human milk contains only 25% of the vitamin K found in cow's milk. Since an intramuscular injection of 1 mg of a thick, yellow vitamin K_1 preparation readily prevents newborn hemorrhage, we include this drug in our routine care of every newborn infant.

Table 6-2 Apgar scoring system of the newborn

	Scoring		
Sign	**0**	**1**	**2**
Color	Blue, pale	Body pink, extremities blue	Pink
Muscle tone	Flaccid	Some flexion of extremities	Well flexed
Heart rate	Absent	⩽100	> 100
Respiratory effort	Absent	Weak, irregular	Good, crying
Reflex irritability (catheter in nose)	No response	Grimace	Cough and sneeze

Resuscitation

Immediately at birth an infant is evaluated according to a plan developed by Dr. Virginia Apgar. The Apgar score uses a point system. Table 6-2 lists the conditions evaluated and shows the basis for assigning points. Infants are given a 1-minute and then a 5-minute Apgar score, with 10 being the highest possible score and 0 being the lowest. If a pale, limp newborn's condition indicates a major difficulty in breathing (Apgar score 0 to 4), he must be put under a warmer with the head and neck correctly extended, the breathing passage must be cleared of secretions, and either an air bag or an endotracheal tube (tube going down the throat into the lungs) should be used to give oxygen.

Oxygen. Oxygen, the life-giving gas we all breathe every moment of our lives, is classified as a drug when used in therapeutic situations. It was discovered in the late 1700s and since then has been used widely to treat breathing problems. Most newborns, even those who are slightly blue around the lips and extremities, do well without it, but asphyxiated infants (those with serious breathing difficulties and low Apgar scores) benefit greatly from oxygen administration. In emergencies, where immediate oxygen treatment is needed, a 5- to 7-liter flow of warmed humidified oxygen should be placed in front of the infant's face. This oxygen is readily available in all delivery rooms from pressurized wall outlets and pressurized cylinders.

Repeated exposure to oxygen can cause a serious eye disease

called retrolental fibroplasia and certain kinds of respiratory problems. However, the importance of minimizing and reversing breathing difficulties at birth far outweighs those potential problems.

Intravenous fluids. Fluids administered by a needle in the veins are often essential when an infant is premature, born to a diabetic mother, small for its age, suspected of being infected, or having severe breathing difficulties. Both water and the simple sugar glucose are very helpful in these critical times because they replace vital fluids and calories lost through excessive urination, breathing, or diarrhea. Glucose is essential for the preservation of the baby's cardiovascular system and central nervous system and for the prevention of low blood sugar levels.

Other drugs. Other drugs are available in case of major problems within the first few hours of life. These must all be used with extreme caution and discrimination because they have numerous side effects. The most important include sodium bicarbonate to counteract excess acid formation in the body; naloxone hydrochloride (Narcan) to counteract the sedating effects of any narcotics given to the mother during labor; epinephrine to stimulate a slow heart rate and increase heart output; atropine to increase heart rate; dopamine to increase heart output; and isoproterenol (Isuprel) for heart stimulation.

■ **Personal experience**

Priscilla S, 38, was a tall, large-boned woman with closely cropped salt and pepper hair and a friendly smile that produced crinkles around her mouth and eyes. She had two children, a girl 5 and a boy 7. Her first pregnancy 9 years ago resulted in a miscarriage. The fourth pregnancy seemed to be going fairly well, although she tired easily, particularly if she were on her feet a lot. She had prominent varicose veins and had to wear elastic stockings from her third month on. Because of her age, her doctors advised her to undergo amniocentesis in the sixteenth week of pregnancy to determine whether the fetus had any genetic defects. Priscilla had A negative blood, and both her children were A positive. Immediately after the delivery of her first two children she had received a shot of RhoGAM to counteract any antibodies she might form against the unborn baby's blood. The physician who had treated her after her miscarriage had had the foresight to give her RhoGAM at that time also. Because of the slight but real danger of maternal-fetal hemorrhage during amniocentesis, Priscilla was given RhoGAM right after the test as a precaution. Four weeks later, to her and her husband's great relief, they found out she was carrying a genetically normal boy.

Priscilla went into labor a week before her due date, and within 3 hours her baby was born. Afterward she hemorrhaged profusely, even after 2 hours of vigorous uterine massage. Her doctor had Pitocin instilled in an intravenous line, and although it caused some heavy cramps, it did help in slowing the flow of blood from her uterus. By the second day post partum her lochial discharge was normal, and she received her RhoGAM injection.

Priscilla's other two children had been bottle-fed babies and had done very well. She decided that she would be more comfortable bottle-feeding her new son also. To stop breast milk production she began taking Bromocriptine tablets in the hospital, and the doctor sent her home with a prescription for the lactation suppressant to last 10 more days. Iron pills were prescribed for a month to replace the iron she had lost during her heavy post-delivery bleeding.

THINGS TO REMEMBER

1. Even though delivery and the postpartum stages of pregnancy are natural and often uncomplicated processes, some medications are necessary to avert certain potentially hazardous complications and to restore the mother to good health as quickly as possible.
2. Oxytocin given intravenously and ergot products given as a pill or injection contract or "shrink down" the uterus to minimize further bleeding. Side effects from these drugs are quite uncommon.
3. Three different forms of breast milk-suppressing drugs are available to mothers not desiring to breast-feed. Each is usually effective, especially if ice packs or breast-binding bras are also used. Side effects are uncommon and can be easily reversed.
4. A pregnant woman whose blood type is Rh negative and is unsensitized is at risk of becoming sensitized to her unborn infant's blood cells if they are Rh positive and cross into the mother's circulation. These persons are eligible for Rh immune globulin in late pregnancy and shortly after delivery (if

the baby's blood type is found to be Rh positive). The intramuscular injection of this drug has led to a dramatic decrease in the incidence of babies found to have red blood cells destruction and severe anemia.

5. Certain disorders of the newborn infant may be prevented by drug treatment after delivery. Silver nitrate or an ointment containing tetracycline or erythromycin is routinely placed in the infant's eyes and lids to prevent serious eye infections, particularly those caused from unsuspected gonorrhea in the mother. An intramuscular injection of vitamin K, which is necessary to enhance the production of certain blood clotting factors, should decrease the chance of bleeding problems in newborn infants.
6. Most newborn infants tolerate the transition from inside to outside the womb very well. Those infants who have breathing problems or difficulties in metabolism usually require supplemental oxygen and intravenous fluids with glucose. If the infant is seriously ill, additional resuscitative efforts are necessary, and they often require potent drugs.

7 Breast-feeding and Drugs

Breast-feeding is very popular and has been on the rise since the middle 1960s. In some communities it is difficult to find a formula-fed baby. The upsurge in breast-feeding coincides with the natural foods and holistic health movement of the last decade and growing public sentiment against artificial products of any sort. Psychologists and pediatricians have demonstrated the importance of the maternal-infant bond in the early days of life and emphasized the role that breast-feeding plays in this bonding process.

The idea is now emerging that breast-feeding provides not only the infant but also the mother with a great deal of sensual pleasure. It may very well be this pleasurable aspect that has helped perpetuate breast-feeding in human cultural evolution. Nursing an infant publicly is considered less negatively than it was 20 years ago. It is a more convenient way of feeding a baby because there is no fuss with bottle and formula preparation and no cleaning up. Nursing is much cheaper than buying formula, so it should be especially attractive to families with limited incomes. Ironically, it seems to be more popular in affluent families.

From both the obstetrician's and pediatrician's point of view, there is no longer any doubt that breast-fed babies are healthier. They have fewer infections, allergies, and digestive upsets. Some researchers have suggested that they exhibit fewer problems with obesity, nervous system development, dental deformities, and learning disabilities. It is not surprising that breast-fed babies do better. Breast milk is perfectly adapted to the needs of the human infant and very different in composition from cow's or goat's milk. It provides food for the baby and takes over where the placenta left off. In some cultures breast milk is called "white blood," an accurate term if you consider that it contains antibodies against all kinds of infections, enzymes that destroy bacteria, virus-inhibiting substances, lactose (milk sugar), which promotes the growth of necessary, helpful bacteria in the intestines, and growth-stimulating molecules that assist the development of cells lining the infant's intestinal tract. Human breast milk has a high concentration of fat and lactose compared with cow's milk, which has a much higher protein component. Milk proteins are casein and whey: in cow's milk casein is the predominant protein; in human milk whey predominates, and it is much easier to digest, especially for small infants.

Substances that enter breast milk

Almost everything the mother eats, drinks, and even breathes will find its way into breast milk. This includes undesirable materials, such as drugs, chemicals, dangerous minerals such as lead or mercury, and environmental pollutants. Physicians are conducting ongoing research on the action of drugs in breast milk and how they transfer to and affect infants. At the moment, however, we do not know a great deal; much of our information comes from reports on studies of one or two patients. We are aware that infants in the first 2 months of life are not equipped to digest or metabolize drugs the way an older child can; therefore certain drugs may accumulate to undesirably high levels in their tiny bodies. Others may simply be excreted with little or no side effects. Each drug behaves in its own unique fashion.

Because mothers are concerned about the effect of pollutants, chemicals, and drugs on their babies, they frequently ask their doctors if breast-feeding should be curtailed if medication is being taken. They also want to know which drugs are safe to take and if breast-feeding ought to be discontinued for short periods after a drug has been swallowed. In most cases the concentrations of drugs in breast milk are low enough that a mother need not stop breast-feeding, unless her baby shows definite symptoms of being affected by the drug. Table 7-1 outlines the effects on the infant of drugs in the mother's breast milk.

Table 7-1 Drugs in breast milk and any effects on the baby*

Drug	Effect on infant at maternal therapeutic doses
Analgesics and antiinflammatory drugs	
Acetaminophen	Detoxified in liver; avoid during immediate postpartum period; otherwise NS†
Aspirin	Transfer to milk not favored; at maternal dose of 12 to 16 tablets per day, no ill effects on infant; When mother requires high antiarthritic doses, monitor infant for bruise potential; may interfere with infant's platelet function
Codeine	NS
Indomethacin (Indocin)	Case report of convulsions in breast-fed infant; used to close patent ductus arteriosus; insufficient data on effect on other vessels; may be toxic to kidneys
Meperidine (Demerol)	NS
Propoxyphene (Darvon, Darvocet)	Only symptoms detectable would be failure to feed and drowsiness; if mother ingests maximum dosage in a 24 hr period, infant could receive 1 mg/day (significant dosage in a neonate)
Antiasthma drugs	
Theophylline	Usually not significant; some reports of irritability and insomnia in infant; caution with sustained-release theophylline products; avoid nursing at time of peak serum level
Terbutaline	NS
Antibiotics	
Ampicillin	NS; possibility of allergic sensitization exists; can produce candidiasis ("thrush," yeast infection) and diarrhea in infant
Cefoxitin (Mefoxin)	NS
Clindamycin (Cleocin)	NS
Erythromycin (Ilosone, E-Mycin)	Use not recommended due to its ability to concentrate in milk; principally excreted in liver; infant's liver function not fully developed: risk of jaundice
Gentamicin (Garamycin)	Not well absorbed from GI tract; may change gut flora; if GI inflammation or diarrhea exists, monitor infant's serum levels to prevent ear and kidney toxicity
Isoniazid	If mother has active tuberculosis, breast-feeding contraindicated; monitor signs of isoniazid toxicity

Modified from Gardner, D.K., and Rayburn, W.F.: Drugs in breast milk. In Rayburn, W.F., and Zuspan, F.P., editors: Drug therapy in obstetrics and gynecology, Norwalk, Conn., 1982, Appleton-Century-Crofts.

*NOTE: Virtually any drug will cross into the breast milk, but the concentration is usually considerably lower than in the mother's bloodstream.

†*NS,* No significant effect.

Continued.

Table 7-1 Drugs in breast milk and any effects on the baby—cont'd

Drug	Effect on infant at maternal therapeutic doses
Antibiotics—cont'd	
Metronidazole (Flagyl)	Contraindicated due to possibly carcinogenic effect (in animal studies) and high milk concentrations
Nitrofurantoin (Macrodantin)	NS, except in G6PD-deficient infant
Nystatin (Mycostatin)	None
Penicillin benzathine	NS; possibility of allergic sensitization
Penicillin G	NS; possibility of allergic sensitization
Penicillin VK	NS; possibility of allergic sensitization
Sulfisoxazole (Ganstrisin)	Watch for jaundice
Anticoagulants	
Heparin	None
Warfarin (Coumadin)	NS; may safely breast-feed; monitor clotting studies
Anticonvulsants	
Carbamazepine (Tegretol)	A 4 kg infant would receive approximately 0.5 mg/kg, which is pharmacologically insignificant
Ethosuximide (Zarontin)	No specific data
Phenobarbital	Maternal doses of 60 to 200 mg/day usually safe for infant; May induce liver enzymes; drowsiness in some cases
Magnesium sulfate	Levels in breast milk increase modestly over the first or second day and return to normal by day 3; calcium levels are unaffected
Phenytoin (Dilantin)	Usually no effect at maternal dosage of 300 to 600 mg/day; possibility of enzyme induction; one case report of a hemoglobin disorder and cyanosis in infant whose mother was taking phenytoin and phenobarbital
Primidone	Drowsiness and decreased feeding; may cause bleeding; avoid use during lactation
Antihistamines and decongestants	
Dexbrompheniramine maleate, 6 mg, with *d*-isoephedrine, 120 mg (sustained-release tablets) Drixoral)	One case report of irritability, excessive crying, and disturbed sleeping patterns of 5 days' duration; avoid long-acting preparations; best to avoid long-acting sustained-release products
Diphenhydramine (Benadryl)	NS; may cause sedation, decreased feeding, or may produce stimulation and rapid heart rate
Cardiovascular drugs	
Digoxin (Lanoxin)	Due to large volume of distribution, total daily excretion of digoxin in mothers with therapeutic serum concentrations would not exceed 1 to 2 *mg* (amount not sufficient to affect child)
Hydralazine (Apresoline)	Jaundice, low platelet count, electrolyte disturbances possible

Table 7-1 Drugs in breast milk and any effects on the baby—cont'd

Drug	Effect on infant at maternal therapeutic doses
Cardiovascular drugs—cont'd	
Methyldopa (Aldomet)	No specific report
Propranolol (Inderal)	NS at dosages up to 160 mg/day
Quinidine	Arrhythmias may occur
Reserpine	May cause nasal stuffiness, lethargy, diarrhea, increased upper airway secretions with difficulty breathing
Diuretic/antihypertensive agents	
Chlorothiazide (Diuril)	Risk of dehydration and electrolyte imbalance; monitor weight and wet diapers and occasional urine specific gravity and serum sodium to ensure status of infant; risk, however, is extremely low; may suppress lactation due to dehydration of mother
Furosemide (Lasix)	None
Hydrochlorothiazide (Hydrodiuril)	Same precautions as chlorothiazide
Gastrointestinal drugs	
Bisacodyl (Dulcolax)	NS
Milk of magnesia	NS
Psyllium hydrophilic mucilloid (Metamucil)	None
Heavy metals	
Iron	Intake of iron is beneficial to mother and infant
Hormones and synthetic substances	
Ethinyl estradiol	Not significant if daily dose is 50 *mg* or less
Mestranol	Not significant if daily dose is 50 *mg* or less
Progestins (19-nortestosterone derivatives)	Not significant if maternal daily dose is 2.5 mg or less
Norethindrone	
Norgestrel	
Norethindrone acetate	
Norethynodrel	
Insulin	Destroyed in infant's GI tract
Prednisone	Long-term effects unknown; minimum amount in breast milk not likely to cause effect on infant in short course
Psychoactive substances	
Amitriptyline (Elavil, Endep)	Probably NS, but long half-life not taken into consideration; watch for depression or failure to feed
Imipramine (Tofranil)	NS at this level; unknown at maternal therapeutic blood levels
Alcohol	Not significant in moderation; lethargy and prolonged sleeping when mother consumes excessive amounts

Continued.

Table 7-1 Drugs in breast milk and any effects on the baby—cont'd

Drug	Effect on infant at maternal therapeutic doses
Psychoactive substances—cont'd	
Barbiturates	NS
Chlordiazepoxide (Librium)	Amount secreted usually insufficient to affect infant, although central nervous system depression has been reported
Diazepam (Valium)	Reports of lethargy and weight loss; infant most susceptible during first 4 days of life; jaundice; most sources do not advise its use during breast-feeding; drug accumulation may occur
Caffeine	Accumulates when intake moderate and continual; causes jitteriness, wakefulness, and irritability
Dextroamphetamine (Dexedrine)	NS; avoid long-acting preparations
Flurazepam (Dalmane)	Some sedation, usually not significant
Marijuana	Conflicting reports; use not recommended; no beneficial effect
Chlorpromazine (Thorazine)	NS at dosages up to 1200 mg/day
Prochlorperazine (Compazine)	None known
Thioridazine (Mellaril)	None known
Trifluoperazine (Stelazine)	None known
Radiopharmaceuticals and diagnostic materials	
Iodine 131	Breast-feeding contraindicated after large therapeutic dose, and should be withheld for 24 hr minimum after smaller diagnostic doses; check milk prior to resuming feeding
^{131}I-labeled macroaggregated albumin	Discontinue breast-feeding for 10 to 12 days, extreme avidity for iodine by thyroid of young infants

Drugs commonly taken while nursing

Alcohol

Almost every source of information dealing with the presence of alcohol in breast milk recounts a particular case report published in 1936 in the medical literature. A mother drank a bottle of port wine over a 24-hour period. Her baby was unarousable from sleep, snored, breathed slowly and deeply, and showed no reaction to pain. This tale may be enough to frighten nursing mothers into complete abstention from alcohol. However, moderate social drinking (two or three cocktails, glasses of wine, or bottles of beer) will produce insignificant effects on the baby. Mild sedation can occur in infants whose mothers have con-

Table 7-1 Drugs in breast milk and any effects on the baby—cont'd

Drug	Effect on infant at maternal therapeutic doses
Radiopharmaceuticals and diagnostic materials—cont'd	
Iopanoic acid (Telepaque)	No adverse effects; iodine excretion can cause rash; probably no problem with just one dose
Tuberculin test	Tuberculin-sensitive mothers can passively immunize their infants through breast milk; immunity may last several years
Thyroid drugs	
Methimazole (Tapazole)	Infant could receive 7% to 16% of maternal dose; could interfere with thyroid function; inhibits synthesis of thyroid hormone
Propylthiouracil	Infant could receive 0.5 mg/day at maternal dosage of 600 mg/day; thought to be harmless; infant could ingest 0.07% of mother's daily dose
Levothyroxine (Synthroid)	May delay clinical symptoms of congenital hypothyroidism in nurslings; improves milk supply in hypothyroid mothers; not contraindicated
Vaccines	
DPT vaccine (diphtheria, polio, tetanus)	NS; does not interfere with immunization schedule
Poliovirus vaccine	Live virus taken orally; not necessary to withhold nursing 30 minutes before and after dose; provide booster after infant no longer nursing
Rubella virus vaccine	No harm but will not confer passive immunity
Hepatitis vaccine	Likely no harm

sumed about eight or nine drinks. Also, this is probably the most a woman could drink and still be conscious enough to nurse her child. There is no evidence that occasional, moderate drinking harms the baby. Obviously, a heavy drinker or chronic alcoholic should not be nursing.

Europeans hold a somewhat more permissive point of view about drinking and breast-feeding. In The Netherlands, for example, physicians encourage the drinking of dark beer for lactating women to promote the production of breast milk. Most physicians and nurses in this country believe that drinking liquids, regardless of whether they contain alcohol, is the most important nutritional factor in good breast milk production.

Caffeine

Although the concentration of caffeine in breast milk is extremely low, it is one drug that can accumulate in the infant's body. If a nursing mother drinks six to eight cups of caffeine-containing beverages (coffee, tea, or colas) per day, her baby is likely to show signs of caffeine stimulation such as hyperactivity and wakefulness. We recommend that nursing mothers limit their intake of caffeine-containing beverages to no more than one or two cups or glasses per day. Many caffeine-free coffees, teas, and colas are available in the supermarket today. (It is interesting to note that there seems to be less reason for concern about caffeine consumption during pregnancy than during nursing, whereas the opposite is probably true for alcohol consumption.)

Cigarette smoke

Nicotine reaches very low levels in breast milk. It is not easily absorbed by the infant's intestines and is metabolized quickly. We do not worry a great deal about infants being poisoned by nicotine received through breast milk, but nicotine does have an impact on breast milk production. Women who smoke 20 to 30 cigarettes per day may produce significantly less milk than their infant needs, causing their baby to have nausea, vomiting, diarrhea, and abdominal cramping. It is worth mentioning also that babies of parents who smoke sometimes have more respiratory difficulties, such as irritation and infection of the lungs, asthma, and other types of allergies.

Painkillers

Aspirin and acetaminophen in normal doses do not appear to affect a breast-feeding infant. If the mother takes the much larger antiarthritis doses of aspirin, there is a risk of interfering with the baby's blood-clotting mechanisms.

Narcotics such as morphine, codeine, meperidine, and methadone do not reach high levels in human breast milk and do not appear to affect nursing infants. Mothers addicted to heroin can be maintained on 50 to 80 mg of methadone per day and still breast-feed their babies.

Propoxyphene (Darvon) may be inadvisable during nursing if the maximum doses are being taken by the mother. One infant was reported to have unusually poor muscle tone when his mother was taking propoxyphene every 4 hours on a regular basis.

Antibiotics

Most antibiotics appear in breast milk, and their concentration depends mainly on their particular chemical properties. Rare reactions to the presence of sulfas in milk have been reported. Penicillins and cephalosporins (Keflex, Ceclor) also maintain low concentrations in breast milk. An allergic reaction has been reported in an infant whose mother was being treated for syphilis with penicillin. This reaction is highly unlikely to occur. Even women who develop breast infections while nursing can normally continue breast-feeding concurrently with antibiotic therapy, unless a severe abscess develops.

Tetracycline should never be taken during pregnancy because it stains the infant's teeth brown. Although there are no reports of this happening during breast-feeding, there is still a theoretical possibility that it could, so an alternative to tetracycline is probably wise.

The aminoglycoside antibiotics (gentamicin, clindamycin) are generally considered safe during breast-feeding because they are not well absorbed through the intestinal tract. If the baby has a gastrointestinal inflammation or diarrhea, he may absorb the drug more efficiently, in which case side effects from the drug might occur. As far as we know, this is only a hypothetical problem.

Chloramphenicol reaches higher levels in breast milk than do many other antibiotics. It should not be used right after birth because it can interfere with bone marrow production in the baby. Some antibiotics concentrate in breast milk in higher levels than in the mother's blood. These include erythromycin, metronidazole (Flagyl), isoniazid, and trimethoprim (Bactrim, Septra). Isoniazid is typically given to individuals with tuberculosis in combination with one or two other drugs. Mothers with active tuberculosis should not be breast-feeding; babies have a very low resistance to tuberculosis and can contract it readily when in close contact with someone who already has the disease.

Blood thinners

The major anticoagulants (blood thinners) are safe during breast-feeding. Heparin molecules are too large to pass into breast milk. Warfarin (Coumadin), a smaller molecule, reaches very low levels in breast milk, although its effects have been known to cause bruising of the nipple. Bleeding and clotting problems have been associated with phenindione and ethyl biscoumacetate.

Laxatives

The safest laxatives for a nursing mother are the bulk formers, which include bran, cellulose, and psyllium hydrophyllic mucilloid. These go under the trade names of Metamucil and Serutan. Milk of magnesia also seems to be safe and does not enter the mother's bloodstream or her breast milk. Stool softeners like dioctyl sodium sulfosuccinate (Colace) are also safe, since they are not absorbed into the mother's system.

The stronger cathartics such as senna, cascara sagrada, danthron, and casanthranol may appear in breast milk and should be avoided if at all possible.

Birth control pills

The hormones found in birth control pills do reach breast milk in very low concentrations. Pill usage during breastfeeding has the potential to decrease the milk supply, change the composition of the milk, and create some undesirable side effects in the baby. If birth control pill use is resumed after an adequate milk supply has been established—usually 1 or more weeks after delivery—it is less likely to influence milk production.

Ten or 15 years ago, when the dosage of hormones in contraceptive pills was much higher, babies had more problems. These included changes in the vagina of baby girls, unusual breast development in boys, and excessive production of bilirubin, a byproduct of liver metabolism. Today, with the low-dosage birth control pills such as Brevicon, Modicon, Lo/Ovral, and Ortho-Novum 1/35, we see fewer problems with milk production and no apparent long-term hazards to the children.

Our preference is to keep our patients from using birth control pills while they are nursing, if they can use another form of contraception satisfactorily. If this is not possible, then the pills should not be taken until 1 week after delivery.

Personal experience

Glenda L was pregnant for the first time at the age of 31. She quit her job as a cashier in the fourth month of pregnancy because she was having backaches. She said, "I just wanted to take it easy and be a housewife for a little while." She gained 40 pounds during her pregnancy, and the doctors predicted that she would bear a large child. Glenda herself was a petite 5 feet 2 inches, and before pregnancy she had weighed 110 pounds. Her baby was due in September, so her pregnancy stretched over the entire summer, including the hay fever season. She had always had problems with allergies, and her pregnancy seemed to make her condition worse than ever. She took Dristan and Allerest, and finally her doctor prescribed Ornade, an antihistamine, to relieve her severe congestion.

After she spent more than 30 hours in labor, Glenda's doctor realized that the baby's head was too large to come through the pelvis, and she decided to perform a cesarean section. After administering epidural anesthesia, she delivered a healthy 9-pound 2-ounce boy. After the operation Glenda began to run a fever and experienced a great deal of pain in her pelvic region. Her doctor suspected a pelvic infection and prescribed two intravenous antibiotics, penicillin and gentamicin. She took Tylenol with codeine every 6 hours or so to relieve her pelvic pain. Finally, because it was still the height of the hay fever season, Glenda had to continue taking Ornade.

Glenda very much wanted to nurse her baby, but she was deeply concerned that the number of drugs she was taking would enter her breast milk and harm her baby. She told the obstetrical nurses that she thought the baby ought to receive formula, but they reassured her that, in spite of her medications, her baby could still be nursed safely. She went ahead with breast-feeding, and the baby suffered no apparent ill effects.

Before her pregnancy Glenda had used birth control pills for contraception. She wanted to resume using them as soon as possible, but her doctor persuaded her to wait until she was through nursing, even though a low-dose pill would probably be safe. She was fitted with a diaphragm and instructed about its use at her 6 weeks postpartum checkup.

THINGS TO REMEMBER

1. The vast majority of drugs a nursing mother would be likely to take do get into breast milk. Most of the time the levels of drugs in breast milk are very low and do not affect the baby.
2. Drugs prescribed for specific medical disorders should be continued because, as in pregnancy, the mother's good health is highly important to successful breast-feeding.
3. A few drugs tend to accumulate in infants because they have immature digestive and excretory systems. These drugs should be avoided. They include erythromycin, metronidazole, trimethoprim, tetracycline, and chloramphenicol when several daily doses are necessary.
4. Most of the drugs commonly used by nursing mothers should not prevent her from breast-feeding. The advantages of breast-feeding usually outweigh any drug effects on the baby.
5. If a baby shows definite symptoms of being affected by a drug and the mother cannot discontinue it or find an acceptable drug substitute, careful scheduling of nursing and drug-taking should be tried. The mother can express milk to be put in bottles or a formula can be substituted when the levels of drug in her bloodstream are likely to be high. Only as a last resort should a mother stop nursing because she must take a drug. The most advantageous time to take a drug when breast-feeding is just before nursing begins, since gastrointestinal absorption takes several hours.

8 Birth Control Pills

Only since 1960 have women had a form of contraception at their disposal that is nearly 100% reliable. The development and marketing of the first birth control pill changed the course of social history because it gave women nearly complete control over their reproductive lives. It is no coincidence that the so-called sexual revolution and the availability of birth control pills started at the same time, and the women's liberation movement followed soon after.

Currently oral contraceptives, also known as birth control pills or just "the pill," are the most popular reversible contraceptive method in the world. In developed countries such as the United States, Canada, The Netherlands, New Zealand, West Germany, and Australia 25% of women of reproductive age are taking the pill. An estimated 5% to 10% of women in the third world countries use oral contraceptives, and their use is increasing.

What is the pill?

Millions of women swallow their pills each day, but what exactly are they taking? To understand how the pill works, an understanding of what happens during a normal menstrual cycle is necessary. Two naturally produced hormones regulate the menstrual cycle—estrogen and progesterone. In the portion of the monthly cycle before ovulation (production of the egg), the estrogen hormone is in charge. After the egg has been released from the ovary into the fallopian tube, it finds its way down into the womb and progesterone takes over. The secretion of progesterone for the next 14 days causes the lining of the uterus to

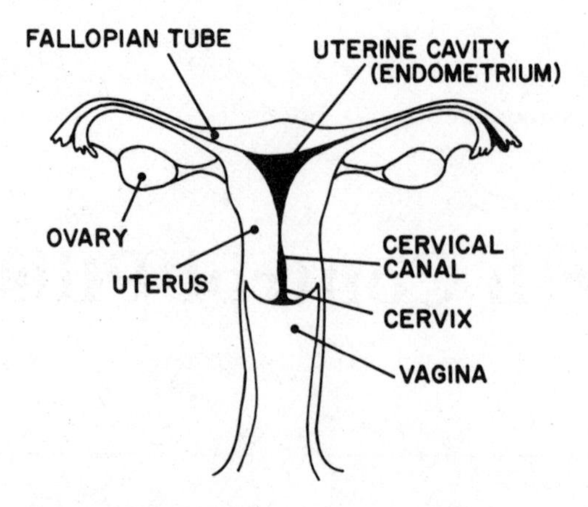

FIG. 8-1 Female reproductive organs.

become thicker. During this time the ratio of estrogen and progesterone changes each day, with progesterone levels mounting as the day approaches when menstruation begins. The lining sloughs off at the end of the cycle as progesterone is withdrawn. The resulting menses lasts for about 5 days, and then the entire process starts over again with estrogen secretion. Fig. 8-1 illustrates the anatomy of the uterus, cervix, and vagina, where the menstrual cycle takes place.

Oral contraceptives attempt to simulate much of the normal menstrual cycle, but prevent conception by suppressing the normal production of estrogen and progesterone by the ovaries. Each oral contraceptive pill combines a synthetic estrogen and a synthetic progesterone called progestin. The synthetic estrogen has two forms, ethinyl estradiol and mestranol.

Under natural conditions estrogen and progesterone are secreted by the ovary and pass directly into the general blood circulation of the body. The hormones contained in oral contraceptives must be absorbed by the intestines, pass through the circulation of the liver, and then enter the general circulation of the body where they can do their work. For the synthetic hormones to work on the reproductive organs, the amount swallowed in the pills must be at least five times higher than what the body would normally produce. This is because most of the synthetic hormones in the pills are broken down by the liver and are not used by the reproductive organs.

Differences between the natural hormone secretion cycle and the synthetic hormone cycle of the pill are as follows: 1. The synthetic hormones enter the body through the intestines and then the liver, whereas natural hormones go into the general circulation directly. 2. The ratio of estrogen to progestin is constant with the pill; the ratio of natural hormones varies. 3. With the pill, estrogen and progestin are administered together, but natural hormones are secreted more or less separately by the ovary.

Effects on the reproductive organs

Oral contraceptives affect the reproductive process in many ways. The pill suppresses the stimulating hormones released from the brain reproductive centers known as the hypothalamus and pituitary gland. This suppression causes the ovaries in women taking oral contraceptives to become small and inactive. The uterus changes also, becoming softer, larger, and slightly bluish. The lining of the uterus, called the endometrium, often is affected to the point where the menstrual flow becomes scanty. If her period stops altogether, a woman is usually advised to refrain from taking the pill to let her uterus and lining regain their normal capacities.

The cervix—the opening of the uterus—is also very sensitive to the effects of synthetic estrogen and progestin. It too sometimes becomes soft and bluish, and cervical mucus changes to a consistency that is nearly impenetrable to sperm. The opening of the cervix sometimes becomes irregular in shape when oral contraceptives are used, but no definitive evidence has been found to show that the incidence of cancer of the cervix is any higher in women who take or have taken the pill. A woman may notice that her vagina is drier when she is taking the pill, and she may be more susceptible to certain kinds of fungal infections, such as those caused by *Candida albicans.* The condition of a woman's vagina while she is taking the pill is affected by the particular pill she takes, the amount of sexual activity she engages in, the number of partners she has, and her personal hygiene. If she runs into a problem with chronic vaginal infections, any one of these items might be the cause.

Both when she is pregnant and when she is using birth control pills, a woman's breasts may increase in size and be more tender than they normally are. Nursing mothers who take oral contraceptives, particularly before 4 weeks post partum, may find that their milk flow decreases, and some studies have shown that the composition of milk changes during pill use. For the most part these problems do not occur when the mother is taking low-dose estrogen pills. Interestingly, there is a significantly lower incidence of fibrocystic breast disease in pill users, anywhere from 25% to 80% lower than that found in women who don't take the pill. This common disorder, characterized by small benign tumors that form in the breasts, seems to be associated with a higher incidence of breast cancer. However, irrespective of their apparently positive effect on possible growth of benign tumors, oral contraceptives should not be prescribed to any woman who has or is suspected of having breast cancer.

Many studies are now in progress to determine the effects of accidental use of oral contraceptives early in pregnancy. Some researchers have suggested that the number of miscarriages due to genetic abnormalities is higher in women who were taking oral contraceptives than in nonusers. No information exists to date on whether genetic defects are higher in babies whose mothers accidentally used oral contraceptives early in pregnancy. There are some claims that a slightly higher incidence of congenital heart or limb defects has occurred in babies whose mothers took the pill when pregnant, but at this point we are unable to make any definitive statements. We would certainly not recommend an abortion just because a mother had been using oral contraceptives at the time of conception.

Effects on other organs of the body

The liver

Since the time the pill was first marketed, many discoveries have been made about how oral contraceptives affect the body. As previously mentioned, the liver is strongly affected by the synthetic hormones in the pill. Particularly in cases when a woman already has an underlying liver disorder, jaundice (yellowing of the skin) may appear when she begins taking the pill, since the liver isn't circulating bile properly. Conditions conducive to gallstone formation, if other factors are present also, are sometimes created. Again, we wish to emphasize that most of these complications were reported on before the introduction of low-dose estrogen or mini-pills. When a woman is taking a pill that has the correct ratio of estrogen to progestin for her system, these problems seldom occur.

High blood pressure

High-dose estrogen birth control pills correlate with increased blood pressure. In one carefully monitored study blood pressure increased by an average of 13.5 mm Hg systolic and 6.2 mm Hg diastolic in all pill users. For women with preexisting hypertension, oral contraceptives are not advisable, regardless of the dosage. If there are no other workable choices, a woman with high or higher than average blood pressure should use a combination pill with a low dose of estrogen (0.5 *mg* or less). She should plan to check her blood pressure at home at least weekly and report any upswings to her physician immediately.

Blood clots

The most serious problem seen in pill users is blood clots. The vulnerable areas in a woman's body are the same as those associated with late pregnancy and delivery: the lower legs, the pelvis, and the lungs. Other factors that make the risk of blood clots higher, especially when they occur in conjunction with oral contraceptive use, are overweight, heredity (clots are three times as common in mothers and daughters or sisters), undergoing major surgery, chronic diseases such as diabetes, varicose veins, and immobility. Deep vein thrombosis has been found to be 5⅛ times higher than normal in women who take the pill. This risk can be greatly reduced with the use of low-dose estrogen pills. However, if a woman has or ever had a blood clot, she should not take oral contraceptives. She should discontinue them immediately if she is taking them. Women with varicose veins or superficial thrombophlebitis are best advised not to use oral contraceptives either.

Heart and blood vessel disease

Contraceptive use has been studied intensively in the United Kingdom, and there they have found that the chance of having a stroke (a clot or bleeding in a specific part of the brain) when using oral contraceptives is four times higher than normal, although the overall risk is still very low. Once again estrogen is the apparent culprit, and the risks are lessened if a low-dose pill

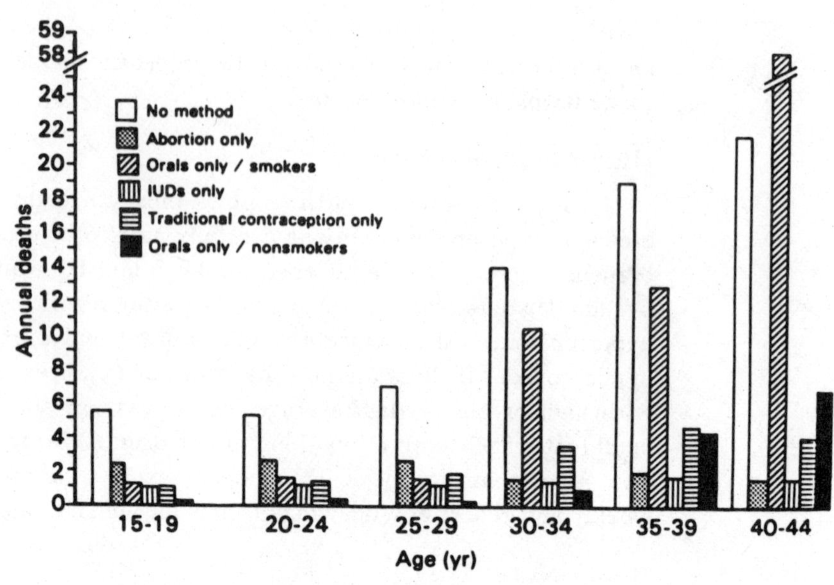

FIG. 8-2 Annual death rate of women associated with the method of birth control used. Note that the risk of death from pregnancy and childbirth with no contraception used is greater than mortality when reversible contraceptive techniques were used, except with oral contraceptive use among women who smoke. (From Tietze, C.: Family Planning Perspectives **9**:74, 1977.)

is being used. If there is a history of stroke in the family, or if a woman has migrainelike headaches or notices a tendency to muscle weakness on one side of her body, she should not use the pill. These all indicate a possible predisposition to stroke.

The risk of a heart attack is significantly higher in women taking oral contraceptives who also have high blood pressure and high levels of fatty substances in their bloodstream. If these women smoke, the risks increase even more and they continue to increase with age. In Fig. 8-2 compare women ages 27 to 39 who smoke and have one incident of heart and blood vessel problems for every 8400 women taking the pill to women ages 40 to 45 who smoke and have one incident of heart or blood vessel problems for every 250 women. Note that in every age group pregnancy is riskier than any given contraceptive method except in women over the age of 40 who smoke. In this group, using the pill is more dangerous than being pregnant.

Who should not use the pill?

From the preceding discussion we can develop a profile of the woman for whom using contraceptive pills is inadvisable. She is 35 years old or older and has been a heavy smoker (1½ to 2 packs of cigarettes per day) for several years. She is 20 pounds or more over the recommended weight for her height and body build. She has one or more of the following medical disorders: high blood pressure, blood clots or a family history of blood clots, high levels of fatty acids in her bloodstream, heart disease of any kind, epilepsy, diabetes, gallstones, or liver disorders. If two or more of these characteristics apply to you, we recommend that you find an alternative to birth control pills. Table 8-1 lists a number of medical problems that make oral contraceptives either inadvisable or absolutely contraindicated.

Probably the two best alternatives to birth control pills are the intrauterine device (IUD) and the diaphragm used in conjunction with contraceptive cream or jelly. The IUD is highly effective in guarding against pregnancy the first year it is in position, with no more than a 1% to 2% pregnancy rate. Complications such as excessive bleeding, cramps, and discomfort sometimes occur, and in such situations the IUD may have to be removed. The optimal time for inserting an IUD is during the first menstrual period after delivery of a baby. An IUD may be inserted immediately after a first-trimester abortion or 2 weeks after a second-trimester abortion.

Diaphragms produce virtually no side effects but are associated with a higher rate of pregnancy (about 13% per year). Most physicians feel this is the result of failure on the part of the user to conform exactly to the requirements of diaphragm usage rather than the result of specific defects of the device. Diaphragms must always be used in conjunction with a spermicidal jelly or cream, which must be reapplied every time intercourse is repeated. The diaphragm should be inserted no more than 6 hours before intercourse and must stay in place at least 8 hours after intercourse has taken place. The diaphragm must be checked periodically for perforations or wear, and it should be refitted if a woman has undergone a weight change of 10 or more pounds or has had a baby.

During the first month of using either the IUD or the dia-

Table 8-1 Conditions in which oral contraceptives are relatively **(R)** or absolutely **(A)** inadvisable to use

Vascular

A 1. Phlebitis—leg vein, pelvic blood clots (i.e., thrombosis)
A 2. Pulmonary embolus—blood clots in lung
A 3. Cerebral vascular accident—stroke
A 4. Coronary occlusion—heart attack
A 5. Blood dyscrasias—leukemia, sickle cell anemia, polycythemia are associated with intravascular blood clotting

Liver

A 1. Jaundice—chronic or recurrent
A 2. Hepatitis—with decreased liver function
R 3. Recurrent pruritus of pregnancy
A 4. Cirrhosis with decreased liver function
A 5. Hepatic porphyria
A 6. Hepatic tumor

Metabolic

R 1. Predisposition to diabetes mellitus
  a. Family history
  b. Family history and obesity
  c. History of large babies (9 lb +)
A 2. Hypertension
  a. Blood pressure 140/90
  b. Previous history of high blood pressure
  c. Black, with family history of high blood pressure
A 3. Lipids
  a. Increased triglycerides
  b. Age 38 or over

Reproductive

A 1. Pregnancy
R 2. Lactation—i.e., nursing
A 3. First degree amenorrhea—i.e., no previous menstrual period
A 4. Second degree amenorrhea—i.e., history of repeated cessation of menstrual periods for 3 or more months *or* chronic infrequent periods
R 5. Second degree amenorrhea and/or lactation while on oral contraceptives—i.e., cessation of menstrual periods and or breast discharge
R 6. Chronic breakthrough bleeding on oral contraceptives—i.e., unpredictable bleeding while on oral contraceptives
A 7. Chronic cystic mastitis in smoker and/or a heavy caffeine user

Miscellaneous concurrent diseases

A 1. Epilepsy
R 2. Migraine headache
A 3. Porphyria
R 4. Fibroid tumors of uterus
R 5. Benign breast tumors
R 6. Varicose veins—severe
R 7. Gallstones or chronic biliary symptoms
A 8. Hyperthyroidism
R 9. Diabetes mellitus

Associated side effects and symptoms

R 1. Chronic weight gain
R 2. Chronic fluid retention
R 3. Chronic gastrointestinal symptoms—nausea, vomiting, dyspepsia
R 4. Chronic premenstrual symptoms—nervous, irritable, depressed, headache, fatigue, lassitude
R 5. Chronic unmanageable leg cramps
R 6. Recurrent vaginal monilial (fungal) infection

From Vorys, N., and Rayburn, W.: Oral contraceptives. In Rayburn, W.F., and Zuspan, F.P., editors: Drug therapy in obstetrics and gynecology, Norwalk, Conn., 1982, Appleton-Century-Crofts.

phragm, a backup contraceptive method such as foam and condom is advisable.

Who may use the pill?

Healthy women under the age of 35 who do not smoke and who maintain a suitable weight for their height and body build should feel confident that birth control pills are a safe and reliable form of contraception, provided that they have not had menstrual problems or other difficulties with their reproductive organs. The pill is an ideal form of contraception for women who want children but plan to postpone their arrival for anywhere from 1 to 5 years. Particularly for those women who feel they would not be able to accommodate a pregnancy for economic, psychological, professional, or any other reason, we recommend the pill because it has the highest rate of effectiveness of all reversible methods available today. It also has the added bonuses of lowering the risks of fibrocystic breast disease and ovarian cancer and cyst formation. Certain menstrual problems such as irregular periods and cramps often improve greatly during and after pill use.

A major drawback of oral contraceptives (if there are no associated medical problems) is cost. They normally run about $9 for 1 month's supply, a price that overstretches the budgets of some women. Planned Parenthood does offer reduced rates on contraceptive materials, and women who are economically strained should visit their local chapters for assistance in purchasing low-cost contraceptives.

Which pill is right for you?

Choosing the right pill is not always easy, and it may be necessary to experiment a little bit before settling on one that can be tolerated for several years. Right now several pharmaceutical houses market at least 27 different compounds. They are prescribed to an estimated 10 million users in North America alone. The major difference among the preparations is the amount of synthetic estrogen or progestin they contain. The range is from 20 to 150 μg of synthetic estrogen and from 0.3 to nearly 10 mg of progestin. Table 8-2 lists some of the popular, currently avail-

Table 8-2 Currently available brands of oral contraceptives

Trade name	Estrogen (μg)	Progestin (mg)
Low dose		
Lo/Ovral	20 Ethinyl estradiol	0.3 Norgestrel
Loestrin 1/20; Zorane 1/20	20 Ethinyl estradiol	1 Norethindrone
Loestrin 1.5/30; Zorane 1.5/30	30 Ethinyl estradiol	1.5 Norethindrone
Ovcon-35	35 Ethinyl estradiol	0.4 Norethindrone
Brevicon; Modicon	35 Ethinyl estradiol	0.5 Norethindrone
Norinyl-1 + 35; Ortho-Novum 1/35	35 Ethinyl estradiol	1.0 Norethindrone
Medium dose		
Norinyl-1 + 50; Ortho-Novum 1/50	50 Mestranol	1 Norethindrone
Ovral	50 Ethinyl estradiol	0.5 Norgestrel
Demulen	50 Ethinyl estradiol	1 Ethynodiol diacetate
Ovcon-50; Zorane 1/50	50 Ethinyl estradiol	1 Norethindrone
Norlestrin 1	50 Ethinyl estradiol	1 Norethindrone acetate
Norlestrin 2.5	50 Ethinyl estradiol	2.5 Norethindrone acetate
High dose		
Ortho-Novum-10	60 Mestranol	10 Norethindrone
Enovid 5 mg	75 Mestranol	5 Norethynodrel
Norinyl-1 + 80; Ortho-Novum 1/80	80 Mestranol	1 Norethindrone
Ovulen	100 Mestranol	1 Ethynodiol diacetate
Norinyl 2 mg; Ortho-Novum-2	100 Mestranol	2 Norethindrone
Enovid-E	100 Mestranol	2.5 Norethynodrel
Enovid 10 mg	150 Mestranol	9.85 Norethynodrel

able brands of contraceptive pills with their dosages of synthetic estrogen and progestin.

Each active tablet contains a specific concentration of estrogen and progestin to be taken daily for 21 days each month. The tablets are packaged in containers that have some sort of calendar to help count the days of use. Some packages contain 28 pills; the last seven pills are inactive, but they are helpful to the user as she counts the days. When taken properly, the pills are nearly 100% effective. Even the very lowest dose pills, which contain only 20 μg of synthetic estrogen, have a pregnancy rate of only 0.2% per 100 women. We advocate using the low-dose compounds because they have fewer side effects and the difference in pregnancy rates is slight.

Getting started on the pill

Choose a doctor who is interested in contraception and who is informed about birth control pills. Before your doctor prescribes a pill for you, he or she will need to know your menstrual and sexual growth history, that is, when you started your periods, developed breasts, etc. You should supply information about any menstrual problems you have had, such as painful or irregular periods. Your general medical history is important too, particularly if you have had some of the health problems discussed previously that can be dangerous when using the pill. Finally, you should have in mind your plans for child-bearing (if you have any) so you can discuss them with your doctor.

Oral contraceptives are prescribed not because a woman is ill, but because she needs a family planning method. Therefore contraceptives should not (1) initiate any new medical problems, (2) aggravate any existing medical condition, (3) allow an unwanted pregnancy to occur, or (4) be associated with dangers to future pregnancies. Because caution is necessary to be sure that none of these things happen, we recommend starting with a low-dose pill (less than 50 *mg* of synthetic estrogen and less than 1 mg of progestin). Higher doses may be necessary if side effects such as no period (withdrawal bleeding) or breakthrough bleeding in between periods occur.

Women will routinely begin a contraceptive pill regimen on the fifth day of their normal period, and the pill should be effective within 2 or 3 days. If periods have been irregular or if the pill wasn't started on the fifth day, a backup method such as a diaphragm should be used with the pill for a full month. Following pregnancy women should wait at least a month or until they have their first period before going back on the pill. If a woman has had a miscarriage or an abortion, she may begin taking the pill within a week if there are no other complications.

If you miss a pill, take two pills as soon as possible. If you miss more than 2 days, begin the pills as soon as possible, but use a backup method for the rest of that monthly pill cycle.

Side effects

Side effects are reported with oral contraceptive usage. A list of common complaints is given in Table 8-3, with advice for man-

Table 8-3 Side effects of birth control pill use

Problem	Recommendations
Acne or unsightly hair growth	Cycle with Ovulen, Norinyl 2 mg, or Demulen
Weight gain	Minimize estrogen/progestin intake (e.g., use Ovcon-35 or Norinyl-1 + 35)
Breast tenderness or enlargement	Use lower dose estrogen/progestin (progestin should be androgenic, e.g., Lo/Ovral or Ovral)
Missed menses	Rule out pregnancy, discontinue pill for 3 months, recycle with higher dose estrogen component
Nipple discharge	Serum prolactin test, rule out pituitary tumor, Pap smear of any unilateral breast discharge, discontinue pill if annoying
Premenstrual tension-like symptoms Fluid retention Nervousness Irritability Headache	Use minimal dose estrogen/progestin, sodium-restricted diet, minimal use of diuretics ("fluid pills")
Vaginal bleeding between menses	Higher dose estrogen/progestin preparation; if continues, discontinue pill
Darker spotting of skin (chloasma)	Use minimal dose estrogen/progestin pill; avoid exposure to sunlight
Nervous symptoms Fatigue Lassitude Decreased sexual desire Mild depression	Use low-dose estrogen/progestin pill; multiple vitamin replacement; pyridoxine, 30 mg 4 times daily
Gastrointestinal symptoms Nausea Vomiting Bloating Itching	Low-dose estrogen/progestin pill; oral cholestyramine and discontinue pill if itching
Yeast infection	Treatment of infection

aging them. Side effects get in the way most during the first 3 months of pill usage. That is why we recommend a 3-month trial before rejecting any particular pill. Women should schedule a visit to the doctor after using the pill for 3 months to make sure there have been no adverse side effects. A yearly office visit is wise, even if there are no apparent problems. During this visit a woman should have a breast examination, a pelvic examination, a blood pressure measurement, an analysis of physical changes such as weight gain, and laboratory blood tests to check the levels of sugars and fats in the bloodstream and the action of blood clotting factors.

The thought of using a drug as potent as the contraceptive pill is upsetting to some women, who will need reassurance and emotional support during their first months of pill usage. Some of the symptoms these women experience may be due merely to nervousness or worry about the consequences of taking the drug. In other cases the woman's symptoms indicate that the proportion of estrogen or progestin should be adjusted. Symptoms that resemble premenstrual distress, such as nausea, nervousness, irritability, water retention, and headaches, probably result from excess estrogen. Symptoms similar to those of pregnancy, like fatigue, sluggishness, depression, increased appetite, and weight gain, may be attributed to too much progestin.

As is true for most drug usage, oral contraceptives may interact with other drugs to produce unanticipated side effects. The desired effect from either the contraceptive or the other drug may not be fully achieved, or undesirable symptoms may occur in the body. Some of the drugs that may reduce the efficiency of contraceptives are the antiseizure drugs phenobarbital, primidone, phenytoin (Dilantin), and ethosuximide; the antibiotics rifampicin and penicillin V; and the sedative and hypnotic benzodiazepines and barbiturates. Drugs whose own activity is affected by the contraceptives include all blood-thinning drugs; insulin and the oral antidiabetic drugs; guanethidine and occasionally α-methyldopa (Aldomet), drugs that control high blood pressure; and all the phenothiazines, including reserpine and the tricyclic antidepressants. In some situations it is possible to modify pill usage to overcome the drug interaction problem; in others it is necessary to discontinue the pill and find an alternate method of contraception.

Morning after pills

Estrogen alone in high doses is a less commonly used type of birth control pill for the "morning after" unprotected intercourse. Changes brought about in the lining of the uterus should prevent sufficient implantation of the fertilized egg. When they were first approved for use about 12 years ago, "morning after pills" were handed out on campuses by student health services and often repeatedly to the same women. Currently, doctors are much more conservative about prescribing a 3- to 5-day trial of these high-dose estrogen compounds because of side effects such as nausea and vomiting. We recommend their use only if absolutely necessary, as in cases of rape, incest, or mechanical failure of a contraceptive. They should not be used repeatedly as a contraceptive technique. High doses of estrogens must be consumed within 72 hours after coitus to prevent pregnancy, and the sooner they are started, the better. Either diethylstilbestrol (DES) or a conjugated estrogen preparation may be used (Chapter 15). The failure rate is about 0.5%, and if the treatment fails or the woman is already pregnant, there is potential for birth defects or tubal pregnancy.

Personal experience

Tracy G first became sexually active in high school, and when she entered college she decided to take birth control pills. Some of her friends in the women's health collective she joined discouraged her, warning that the pills had dangerous side effects and that she was doing things to her body that she probably didn't realize. Nevertheless, Tracy was healthy and wanted to be completely free in her sexual activities. The only contraceptive that offered her that type of freedom was the pill. She started on Norinyl 1 + 35 without difficulty and stayed with it about 9 months. At that time she began to spot between her periods and then she missed a period. Panic-stricken, she went to the doctor, but he explained to her that it was not pregnancy causing her to miss the period, but rather the effects of the birth control pills. Several of her friends said, "I told you so."

The doctor, however, thought that Tracy's problem was that she was not using a pill with a high enough estrogen dosage. He suggested that they give a higher dosage pill a chance, and Tracy agreed to go with pills one more time. She began taking Norinyl 1 + 50. After 3 months she was once again established on a normal menstrual cycle with no spotting and with periods from 3 to 5 days in length. Her blood pressure was normal, but she did put on 3 pounds, which may have been due to fluid retention. Tracy decided that 3 extra pounds were worth the freedom from worrying about pregnancy.

THINGS TO REMEMBER

1. In the 20 years since the birth control pills were first marketed, we have made great progress. We now understand more about the dosages of hormones necessary, and thus the amounts of both estrogen and progestin have been considerably lowered. We have also determined contraindications for usage and medical disorders where the pill should not be used.
2. Oral contraceptives are a safe, highly effective form of birth control when used correctly by healthy, relatively young women with no contraindicative medical problems.
3. With use of birth control pills, women are less likely to have fibrocystic breast disease, breast cancer, ovarian cancer, or menstrual discomfort.
4. Oral contraceptives do have strong effects on both the reproductive system and on other organs of the body. Sometimes women will experience nagging symptoms, especially during the first 3 months of pill usage. If a pill does not work out after a 3-month trial, a woman should visit her doctor to request a different pill or an alternative method of birth control.
5. Usually the lower the dose of estrogen in the pill, the fewer the noticeable side effects. For practical purposes lower dose estrogen pills are just as effective as high-dose estrogen compounds.
6. The pill is risky for women with certain medical problems, such as high blood pressure, blood clots, diabetes, heart or blood vessel disease, epilepsy, liver disorders, or gallbladder problems. Being overweight or smoking increases the hazards from pill usage, especially in women over age 35.
7. The alternatives to pill usage, such as a diaphragm or an IUD, should be carefully considered before the pill is discontinued.
8. It is important to see your doctor regularly when you are taking the pill. You will need a routine examination after the first 3 months of pill usage and annually from then on.
9. Oral contraceptives interact with certain other drugs. Sometimes the effectiveness of the contraceptives will be reduced; at other times the effectiveness of the other drugs will be diminished when the two are taken simultaneously.

Always tell the doctor who prescribes your birth control pills about any other medication you are taking.

10. The "morning after" pill is a high-dose estrogen birth control pill given for 3 to 5 days to prevent implantation of the fertilized egg. It is not to be taken routinely for birth control but is helpful in cases involving rape, incest, or possible failure of a condom, diaphragm, or IUD.

9 Menstrual Irregularities

Most people need to have certain elements in their lives that they can depend on, that are predictable, and that go like clockwork and don't let them down. Many women feel that way about their menstrual periods. A regular monthly cycle is a comfort and an assurance that the body is working well and that life has a certain pattern to it that can be relied on. Thus, when something changes and the menstrual cycle doesn't follow its normal course, it can be very upsetting. Women often respond with fear and anxiety that something bad is happening—a disease, a cessation of their feminine functions, or an unwanted or complicated pregnancy.

First of all, we want to reassure women that almost no one goes through a lifetime of menstruation without some variation in the pattern. This can be caused by any number of things, which do not necessarily mean a problem: a hormone fluctuation, stress or excitement, or a change of diet or environment. Before she starts to worry, a woman should allow herself to go through two or three succeeding menstrual cycles, watching carefully for symptoms and notable occurrences to report to her doctor, if it becomes necessary to see a physician.

A menstrual cycle occurs approximately every 28 days, with normal variations being 7 days more or less. Menstrual flow will generally be moderately heavy on the first 1 or 2 days and then begin to taper off. Again, there is quite a degree of normal variation from woman to woman in the amount of flow, but a moderately heavy menstruation will require a change of pad or tampon about every 2 hours. Most women do not menstruate for less than 3 or more than 7 or 8 days, and 5 days is probably an average length for a period.

When using the term *menstrual irregularities,* we are basically talking about these problems: vaginal bleeding that occurs either too frequently or too infrequently and bleeding that is too light or too heavy.

Frequent or heavy menstrual flow

Perhaps most common and worrisome to a woman is excessive menstrual flow or very frequent uterine bleeding. This usually results from a hormone imbalance with anovulation (failure to produce an egg), but it also occurs because of an ovarian or uterine tumor, as a complication of early pregnancy, or in a bleeding disorder not related to the reproductive system. Women are primarily concerned when their bleeding is heavy, unpredictable, and uncontrollable. This type of hormone-related bleeding is painless and rarely associated with any physical discomfort. It can, however, lead to anemia and great fatigue.

Sometimes, after having a baby, women will experience several weeks of sporadic and unpredictable bleeding. This, too, is hormone related. Ovulation does not usually occur until at least 1 month after delivery. Typically, unless she is breast-feeding, a woman can expect postpartum discharge, or lochia, for a few days to a few weeks after delivery, and then she will revert to a normal menstrual cycle. Breast-feeding often prevents or delays ovulation and the return to a normal menstrual cycle, and women who nurse their babies may have to wait many months before having a normal period. A few women fall into a sort of in-between stage. Nursing prevents the appearance of a full-fledged period, but the ovaries still begin to produce fairly high levels of estrogen, which cause periodic bleeding without ovulation. This is nothing to be concerned about, but contraception is mandatory, since ovulation is likely to occur at almost any time.

How much is too much?

The extent of bleeding may be estimated by recording the number of pads used each day and the degree of pad saturation. If you need to change pads more often than every 2 hours and if your pads are 80% or more saturated, you are probably bleeding excessively. You should have a physical examination to determine where the bleeding comes from: a vaginal laceration, the cervix itself, or the uterus. At that time the doctor may be able to determine any tumors that are growing in your cervix, uterus, or ovaries or any foreign bodies that may be in the reproductive tract. With this examination you should have a Pap smear and a complete blood count. If your symptoms persist without a specific diagnosis, your doctor can consider testing your blood-clotting ability, pituitary gland function, thyroid gland function, and ovarian function. He or she may wish to perform a biopsy (removal of a small piece of tissue) of your endometrium (uterine lining) or cervix.

Therapy

Women visiting the doctor because of excessive vaginal bleeding are often adolescents or are near menopausal age. Between the ages of 12 and 16 the ovaries are frequently not sufficiently stimulated by the hormones from the pituitary gland to release an egg. Ovulation usually begins to occur somewhere between 2 and 5 years after the first menstruation; once it does, irregular bleeding tends to clear up. If it doesn't, the doctor must begin to consider other sources of the problem, and these are listed in Table 9-1. Around the time of menopause, ages 40 to 55, irregular periods are also related to lack of ovulation. Near menopause the function of the ovaries gradually decreases, with a resulting lack of egg production and sex hormones, especially progesterone.

If no other medical disorder is involved and the cause of bleeding is anovulation with consequent hormone imbalance, the primary form of treatment involves the use of supplemental hormones. A woman with heavy active bleeding usually responds to a combination of high-dose estrogens and progestins or a high-dose birth control pill preparation. Either combination taken

Table 9-1 Conditions related to excessive or frequent menstrual bleeding

Lack of ovulation	Stress
Excess weight gain	Underactive thyroid
Early menopause	Polycystic ovaries
Medications	Overactive adrenal glands
Sex hormones	Central nervous system disorder
Tranquilizers	Intrauterine device
Some high blood pressure medications	Cancer of cervix or uterus

four times daily will usually decrease the bleeding within the first 2 days and stop it within 7 days. Intravenously injected estrogens may be necessary to stop uterine bleeding quickly. The dosage of hormone preparation is then usually cut in half for the next 3 weeks. Menstruation should occur within 3 days after termination of drug therapy. Common problems associated with this initial therapy using high-dose hormones are nausea and vomiting. For this reason women over 35 who smoke should take a progestin-only pill because of the increased risk of heart attack associated with high-dose estrogens. The monthly treatment cycle should be continued for 3 cycles: use of the medication for 3 weeks and discontinuation of the drug for a week to allow withdrawal bleeding to occur each month. If the uterine lining becomes very thin after a prolonged period of bleeding, a conjugated estrogen tablet may be necessary to reestablish this lining. When uterine bleeding has stopped or decreased sufficiently, the doctor may prescribe lower dose oral contraceptives so that the period of bleeding may be planned and limited.

Further management

Once a woman's bleeding has come under control after the 4-month drug course, recurrence of the problem depends on whether she resumes egg production. If she does not plan to become pregnant, she can continue taking an oral contraceptive, either a regular dose or low-dose birth control pill or a progestin-only pill. Medroxyprogesterone acetate (Provera), 10 mg per day for 5 days every 2 months, will allow predictable withdrawal bleeding to occur. If regular menstrual cycles begin to occur, hormone pills are no longer necessary. If a woman does wish to become pregnant, she may take a fertility drug instead of a birth control pill. Clomiphene (Clomid), for example, will enhance the release of hormones from the pituitary gland, which stimulates the ovary to produce eggs (Chapter 11).

Bleeding that continues after a course of estrogen therapy as just described may require the doctor to perform a dilatation and curettage (D&C) of the uterus or an endometrial biopsy. This is especially true if a woman is age 35 or older. Other means for evaluating the lining of the uterus include a hysterosalpingogram, in which a dye is injected into the uterus to allow an x-ray view of it, and a hysteroscopy, in which a telescopic instrument is inserted up the vagina, through the cervix, and into the uterus to permit the doctor to see internal structures.

Light or infrequent menstrual flow

For the most part light or infrequent menses are associated with early pregnancy, excessive weight gain, menopause, use of certain drugs, disturbances of the central nervous system, very strenuous exercise, or emotional problems (Table 9-2). Each one of these causes has a different origin and requires specific treatment by a physician or suitably qualified person, particularly if the infrequent or scanty bleeding goes on for several months.

Most women do not mind if the menstrual flow is light or infrequent on occasion. Remember that ovulation and pregnancy still can occur; if you are sexually active, particularly if you are over 40, effective contraceptive techniques are mandatory.

Unless you have a particular medical problem that explains a persistent irregularity or light flow, the most common reason for this to happen is that your ovaries do not produce an adequate amount of estrogen and progesterone. If you decide to have this problem treated with drugs, the therapy should be directed toward stimulating the ovaries using either fertility drugs or estrogen and progestin pills. Fertility pills should be used only if you want to become pregnant and it has been ascertained that lack of ovulation is the cause of your menstrual irregularity.

Most women with scant or infrequent menstrual bleeding do not wish to become pregnant and therefore prefer to take an oral contraceptive or sequential estrogen and progesterone replacement. We usually recommend a conjugated estrogen tablet such

Table 9-2 Conditions related to light or infrequent menstrual bleeding

Pregnancy; ectopic pregnancy	Medications, especially use of low-dose oral contraceptives, cessation of oral contraceptives, or use of long-acting progestin injections
Threatened miscarriage	Lean muscular bodies, strenuous exercise, and high stress
Chronic medical illness	Anxiety, stress, or other emotional problems
Menopause	Drastic weight changes
Lack of ovulation	
Underactive pituitary gland	
Central nervous system disorder	
Scarred or inactive uterine lining	
Genetic disease	

as Premarin in strengths of 1.25 mg. These should be taken each day from days 1 to 24; then a progestin tablet, usually 10 mg of Provera, should be taken from days 20 to 24. Menstruation should begin by day 27 and last for the remainder of the month. This regimen should be adequate not only for regulating periods but also for dependable contraception in most adult women. Adolescents with less sexual development (very small breasts, for example) may benefit from a higher dose estrogen pill, such as conjugated estrogens in strengths of 2.5 mg. At this age side effects from estrogen therapy, such as weight gain, are not very common.

Personal experience

Martha H, a 40-year-old homemaker and mother of three children, had been in good health for years. She had had a tubal ligation 4 years ago, after the birth of her last child. Her only complaint was that she carried around 30 extra pounds on her strong, solid body, and she couldn't seem to get rid of them. Then she began to notice irregularities in her menstrual cycle. Sometimes her periods would come twice in one month and sometimes not at all. Her bleeding had become very heavy, and she found that even when wearing a super tampon and a maxi-pad, she had to change almost every 2 hours. The period she was having when she arrived at her doctor's office had been going on for 2 weeks.

On examination the doctor ascertained that she had a slightly enlarged uterus but found nothing else of note. Her doctor suspected a hormone imbalance and decided to prescribe Provera. She took 10 mg of Provera per day for the first 5 days of her monthly cycle to control when her monthly periods would begin. She also took iron pills because blood tests revealed that she had become anemic.

Two months later Martha reported back to the doctor that she was feeling more capable of dealing with her three lively children and that the amount of blood lost during each period had decreased considerably. Despite this, she continued to have occasional spotting between periods for 6 more months, so her doctor scheduled a D&C. After gently scraping her uterine lining, the doctor discovered a noncancerous endometrial polyp. With the polyp removed, Martha's spotting disappeared, and she stopped taking Provera soon after that. She has had no further menstrual irregularities.

THINGS TO REMEMBER

1. Most women have a strong psychological need for regular and predictable menstrual cycles, and the need to treat irregularities cannot be overemphasized.
2. Abnormal menstrual bleeding is most commonly represented by painless and heavy or more frequent flow. This additional blood loss is often perplexing, since it is usually unpredictable and may be difficult to control.
3. Excessive or frequent uterine bleeding occurs most commonly during adolescence or around menopause. Many physical and psychological conditions are associated with menstrual irregularities, but the most common is lack of ovulation.
4. Your doctor should give you a thorough physical, including a Pap smear. Further testing may be necessary if certain medical conditions, such as a thyroid problem or bleeding disorder, are suspected.
5. Choosing a treatment for excessive vaginal bleeding is not always easy. Unless a medical disorder is found, the doctor will usually prescribe a high-dose estrogen and progestin pill to temporarily correct any hormone imbalance. Once the bleeding has diminished, the problem should be managed with lower doses of the same pills prescribed for 3 weeks out of each month.
6. Surgical procedures such as a D&C or hysterectomy are rarely necessary to begin with, but a D&C at least may be required if bleeding continues after use of the hormone pills. Other procedures, such as a hysterosalpingogram or hysteroscopy, may be performed to visualize the inside of the uterus so the doctor can locate precisely the source of the bleeding.
7. A woman with persistent scanty or infrequent menstrual bleeding should be evaluated by a physician. In many cases her menstrual cycle may be safely regulated with oral contraceptives or a monthly schedule of sequential estrogen and progestin tablets.

10 Menstrual Cramps, Premenstrual Syndrome, and Chronic Pelvic Pain

Almost no women go through their reproductive years (ages 12 to 50) without some episode of lower abdominal or pelvic pain. This discomfort may come and go; it may occur only around the time of the menstrual period; or it can be continuous. Menstrual discomfort is one of the leading causes of absenteeism from school and work. The cash value of time lost on the job, at home, and in the community due to menstrual problems is enormous, in the millions of dollars. The toll it takes on women themselves is immeasurable, but surely very great.

Premenstrual symptoms such as fatigue, backache, abdominal swelling, and "the blues" can be extremely incapacitating. The extent of incapacitation both with cramps and premenstrual syndrome varies greatly and is often unpredictable. Severe symptoms during the week before menstruation have been associated with an increased rate of suicide attempts, acute psychiatric illness, violent crimes, and accidental deaths.

The premenstrual syndrome (PMS) achieved some notoriety in 1982 when a 24-year-old woman from New York City was acquitted of a felonious assault charge; her defense was that it was caused by an acute case of PMS. Whether this legal precedent will work in favor of or against women remains to be seen, but it has certainly opened a new vista on the problems associated with menstruation.

History of menstrual pain treatment

Pain associated with menstruation has challenged physicians throughout the ages. The ancient Greeks described the pain-killing effects of sweet wine, fennel root, and rose oil when applied to the external genitals of menstruating women. Hippocrates, the father of modern medicine, believed that obstruction of the cervix and retaining of menstrual fluids cause painful menstruation. For a long time many physicians agreed with this concept and practiced dilation of the cervix to relieve menstrual pain. Chinese women were treated with moxibustion, a technique in which a cone of wormwood was rolled into what looked like a giant cigarette, placed on a ginger slice at a specific point on the abdomen, ignited, and allowed to burn until the skin became reddened and heated. In the mid 1800s removal of both ovaries became a popular remedy for menstrual distress. At the turn of the century a number of plant extracts and synthetic chemicals were used, with opium being the most popular. Women took nitroglycerine for hot flashes and pale skin.

Not until 1930 did physicians begin to get some idea of what really caused menstrual distress; they noted the connection between menstrual pain and ovulation and shortly after that began to treat dysmenorrhea (painful menstruation) with estrogens. Following their introduction in the late 1950s, oral contraceptives became the favored treatment for menstrual disorders. It wasn't until the mid 1960s that another breakthrough occurred—the discovery of the relationship between prostaglandins and menstrual pain. Prostaglandins are a chemical produced by elements of the nervous system and many other parts of the body and are found in abundance in the uterus. In the early 1970s researchers realized that aspirin and similar compounds inhibited prostaglandin formation. Women had been taking aspirin to relieve menstrual distress for years, and research revealed that it had some effectiveness as a prostaglandin inhibitor. Many new drugs that were developed in the 1970s proved to be much more effective than aspirin. Currently doctors feel that further refinement of these prostaglandin-inhibiting drugs will provide an even better means of controlling dysmenorrhea in the future.

Other types of pelvic pain

Disorders that tend to be long standing or chronic include endometriosis (islands or clusters of glands normally found on the inner surface of the uterus that migrate to and begin growing on the surface of other pelvic organs), ovarian tumors, uterine tumors, adhesions (thin, fibrous bands around the tubes or ovaries from prior pelvic infections or surgery), a backward displacement of the uterus, congestion or engorging of the uterine blood vessels, or persistent infections of the uterus, tubes, and ovaries. Each form of pelvic discomfort represents a different kind of challenge both to the woman and to her doctor.

Menstrual cramps

From time to time most women complain of episodes of dull, intermittent lower abdominal cramps just prior to or during the first few days of their period. The pattern does not appear to change, even after pregnancy, but it does diminish with age.

The uterus is continually contracting, and menstrual cramps are simply stronger, more frequent versions of these same contractions. What causes the contractions to intensify during menstruation? Prostaglandins—the chemicals that researchers linked with pelvic pain almost 20 years ago. Prostaglandins increase their concentration in the uterus after ovulation and reach their peak at the onset of menstruation, after which they are discharged in the menstrual flow. By causing the muscle of the uterus to tighten, the prostaglandins inhibit the oxygen supplied to the uterus through the blood vessels. Any muscle that is deprived of oxygen will be painful and, as menstrual cramp sufferers know only too well, the uterus is no exception.

The discovery of prostaglandins shifted much of the thinking about dysmenorrhea. Before that many individuals, physicians and lay people alike, regarded menstrual pain as a psychological problem as much as a physical one. Now the physical cause of dysmenorrhea is firmly established. Psychological factors cannot be entirely discounted, however, because menstruation is so intimately connected with a woman's sexuality and by extension her relationship with her primary sexual partner or mate. Menstrual cramps caused by prostaglandin production have a fairly specific pattern of occurrence. Usually they start shortly after release of the egg from the ovary and get worse until the menstrual flow begins. They are most intense just before the onset of a period. Menstrual pain that seems more erratic or can be related to emotional upsets may have its roots in psychological disturbance. Of course, diseases often start because of emotional stress but perpetuate themselves because certain physiological processes become established. Situations like these require a dual approach, with both the emotional origins and the current physiological problems being treated.

Many drugs are currently available to relieve the physiologically based symptoms caused by excess prostaglandin production. They act in different ways: to inhibit ovulation, to decrease prostaglandin production, or to slow down the force and frequency of uterine contractions. Side effects from these drugs must be considered along with the relief from menstrual cramping they provide.

Drugs that stop the production or synthesis of prostaglandins are called prostaglandin synthetase inhibitors (PGSIs). They are considered to be effective in 60% to 85% of women. Since prostaglandins are produced in other cells in the body, the PGSIs may prevent their production in other tissues besides the uterus with relief of symptoms such as bowel difficulties, headache, and backache. Certain side effects of these drugs do, however, limit a person's tolerance to them. The PGSI products currently marketed in the United States are listed in Table 10-1. These drugs must be taken when menstrual cramps begin. All require a prescription except, of course, aspirin and acetaminophen. Aspirin and acetaminophen are not as effective in their action on the uterus as are the other PGSIs.

Women often describe severe menstrual cramps as laborlike uterine pains. Sufferers can be treated with the same drugs used to stop premature labor, such as terbutaline, ritodrine, alcohol, or aminophylline. Unfortunately, most of these drugs have side effects that offset their value in relieving menstrual discomfort. For example, some women may use alcohol for temporary relief of cramping and end up being addicted to it after prolonged and excessive use.

Evidence suggests that a deficiency of magnesium accounts for some cases of menstrual cramps. Taking magnesium oxide pills in doses of 100 mg four times per day corrects magnesium deficiency. We suggest that the mineral be taken through two full

Table 10-1 Drugs to treat menstrual cramps and chronic pelvic pain

Drug	Dosage
Indomethacin (Indocin)	25 mg three times per day; 50 mg three times per day
Naproxen (Naprosyn)	250 mg (2 to start); then 250 mg every 4 to 6 hours
Naproxen sodium (Anaprox)	275 mg (2 to start); then 275 mg every 6 to 8 hours
Ibuprofen (Motrin)	400 mg three times per day
Fenoprofen (Nalfon)	200 mg every 4 to 6 hours
Mefenamic acid (Ponstel)	250 mg (2 to start); then 250 mg every 6 hours

menstrual cycles before you decide whether it is the answer to your menstrual cramp problem. Pyridoxine (vitamin B_6) is advocated by some doctors for cramps. Take it in daily doses of 1 to 8 50-mg pills through the entire menstrual cycle. If necessary, increase your intake to 800 mg per day immediately before or during the menstrual period. Magnesium and vitamin B_6 are considered harmless in the dosages we have recommended; on the other hand, their effectiveness is not guaranteed, and more research needs to be done on their role in relieving menstrual pain.

The most useful drugs for relieving menstrual cramps probably are the oral contraceptives. By stopping ovulation (Chapter 11) they prevent the formation of high levels of prostaglandins. The birth control pills that contain high amounts of progestin and low quantities of estrogen are the best to use. A progestin-only pill such as Ovrette, Micronor, or Nor-QD sometimes helps but tends to cause more menstrual irregularities than do pills that also contain estrogen. A woman should allow at least a 3-month trial of any pill she uses for menstrual problem relief before deciding whether it is effective. Understandably, most women are reluctant to take hormone pills for menstrual discomfort unless their problem is severe. The same guidelines that are outlined in Chapter 9 apply in this situation: if a woman is under 35, otherwise in good health, not substantially overweight, and a nonsmoker, she stands to gain much more than she loses by using oral contraceptives to relieve menstrual pain.

Table 10-2 Specific premenstrual symptoms and proposed therapy

Symptom	Treatment
Light-headed (low blood sugar level)	Frequent, small meals
Nausea	Vitamin B_6
Abdominal bloating	Salt restriction
	Spironolactone, 25 mg four times per day 2 weeks before menstruation
Tension	Progesterone, 200 mg rectal or vaginal suppositories
	Bellafoline (Bellergal), 1 tablet three times per day
Tender breasts	Bromocriptine, 2.5 mg two times per day during 2 weeks before menstruation

The premenstrual syndrome

Physical and psychological premenstrual symptoms vary greatly from woman to woman and at different stages in a woman's reproductive life. Some women have no problems, whereas others are incapacitated to the point where they cannot perform even simple daily tasks. Unlike menstrual cramps, premenstrual tension does not have to be preceded by ovulation. Its symptoms include abdominal bloating, swelling of the legs and ankles, backache, breast tenderness, the "blues," crying spells, irritability, fatigue, increased hunger, and weight gain. These complaints are also familiar to pregnant women.

If you suffer from the symptoms of premenstrual syndrome, try maintaining a daily diary of symptoms for at least 2 months. By doing so, you will be able to describe to your doctor how severe specific complaints are and relate them to the time within the menstrual cycle when they occur. Notice if there is a relationship to exercise, dietary habits, family difficulties, or stress at work. It may be that counseling or a search for a medical disorder such as an overactive thyroid is what is really needed. As previously indicated, it is important to gain another perspective if symptoms have no identifiable pattern, do not occur consistently within a few days before menstruation, or persist after menstruation is over.

Drug therapy usually aims toward relief of one or two of the more uncomfortable symptoms of premenstrual syndrome (Table 10-2). Since a single specific cause to explain this wide range of symptoms remains more theoretical than real, drugs are not always successful. Vitamin B_6 may be given for at least 2 months in daily doses of 50 mg, with increases up to 800 mg per day if relief does not occur. Ironically, certain side effects of vitamin B_6, such as nausea, headache, and the blues, duplicate the symptoms of the very problem it is attempting to relieve. We advise against the use of antidepressants or tranquilizers like chlordiazepoxide (Librium) or diazepam (Valium) for premenstrual tension. Emotional support, sensitive counseling, and education are often much more effective. Many women take fluid pills (diuretics) to guard against weight gain and swelling. Diuretics are basically harmless, but if a woman uses them for a prolonged period she may wash certain important chemicals like sodium or potassium out of her body. This is called an electrolyte imbalance, and it can create unpleasant symptoms: dizziness, fainting, weakness, and extreme fatigue. Once again, birth control pills are the only drugs that have helped large numbers of women with premenstrual symptoms. By putting the ovaries to rest, the production of estrogen and progesterone is decreased, and the problem is at least temporarily eliminated.

Chronic pelvic pain

A large proportion of women visiting gynecologists seek relief from pelvic pain that has been present for months or even years. If you have this problem, your doctor will need to take a thorough history to find out if your pain has been continuous or intermittent, where it is located, how it relates to urination and bowel movements, whether you have had any vaginal infections, if it occurs during sexual activity, and how it relates to different kinds of stress in your life. Along with a review of your past medical, obstetrical, and surgical history, he or she will perform a complete abdominal and pelvic examination. Findings may include a mass in the lower side, which could be an ovarian cyst, ovarian tumor, fallopian tube abscess, endometriosis, or stool in the bowel; tenderness on moving the uterus, which could be infection, excess scar tissue from previous surgery, or endometriosis; enlarged uterus, which could be adenomyosis, pelvic congestion, or fibroid tumors; or backward displacement of the uterus, which could represent adhesions or the "universal joint syndrome." If no abnormalities are apparent, we recommend an observation period of 3 to 6 months during which an antibiotic such as penicillin, a PGSI, or a mild painkiller should be taken.

When is surgery necessary?

Pelvic pain is one of the most frustrating complaints physicians encounter, and they often have difficulty evaluating and controlling it. Diagnostic surgery becomes necessary if an obvious pelvic mass persists or if a woman cannot obtain relief from medicines.

During surgery, while the person is fully anesthetized, the doctor performs a thorough pelvic examination. If no obvious problem surfaces, he or she usually dilates the cervix and lightly scrapes the uterus. This is the well-known D&C (dilatation and curettage). A laparoscope, a long, tubelike, telescopic instrument, is then inserted just below the navel to permit the doctor to actually see the ovaries, tubes, uterus, and outside walls of the bladder and bowel. At this time the doctor can obtain fluids for culture of any infectious organisms or a piece of tissue for biopsy or break up any scar tissue that might be causing problems.

Sometimes the source of the pelvic pain will be unveiled during exploration with the laparoscope, and more extensive surgery or stronger drug therapy will be indicated. It is quite appropriate to ask your doctor to explain the laparoscopic findings to you, using nontechnical terms and drawings if necessary.

If no solution is immediately forthcoming, then the search must continue, with perhaps another trial period of medications or further examination of problems such as sexual dysfunction, marital discord, fears, or phobias. We do not believe that the nerves which carry pain from the pelvic region should be severed or that organs like the uterus or ovaries should be removed just because no other answer can be found. Occasionally an injection of local anesthetic through the vagina and into the cervix may help you with acutely painful episodes. Hypnosis, biofeedback, and relaxation techniques have also been used with varying degrees of success.

■ Personal experience

Erin C, a small, serious 22-year-old graduate research assistant, has had nearly incapacitating menstrual cramps since the age of 13. Her large brown eyes reflected pain as she described the nausea, cramping, bloating, and extreme frustration she experienced with each menstrual period. For years she used aspirin to relieve the pain associated with her period, but it was not terribly helpful. Recently she had been given Ponstel by a gynecologist whom she had since stopped seeing. She found the Ponstel to be more helpful than aspirin, but it by no means solved her problem.

A pelvic examination revealed only a vague tenderness and feeling of fullness near her right ovary. Erin's new doctor suggested birth control pills to see if they would help her menstrual discomfort. She refused, afraid of subjecting her body to synthetic hormones.

Six months later Erin was at her doctor's office again. In the time that had elapsed she had become sexually active, and much of the time found intercourse to be quite painful. Determined to get to the bottom of her problem, she asked her doctor if she would perform exploratory surgery, and she reluctantly agreed. With Erin under general anesthesia, the doctor looked into her abdomen with a laparoscope. Around the bladder and the ligament near the right ovary and tube she saw a suspicious "powder burn" area, suggesting endometriosis. When Erin had recovered from the anesthesia, her doctor sat down with her and explained that a low-dosage oral contraceptive might go a long way in relieving her menstrual distress and preventing the endometriosis from spreading. She agreed to start taking Brevicon.

During the subsequent year her pain faded considerably, and she found sexual intercourse to be much more enjoyable. She decided to take Brevicon for another year, not only for the pain relief it offered her but also because of its contraceptive effects.

THINGS TO REMEMBER

1. Recurring or persistent pelvic pain is a common reason for a young or middle-aged woman to be absent from school or work and to ultimately seek medical attention.
2. The relationship of pain and other premenstrual symptoms to the menstrual cycle is important to determine. Before visiting the doctor you should keep a daily diary of these symptoms, noting when they occur, what they occur in conjunction with, and what relieves or worsens your discomfort.
3. At present, the prostaglandin synthetase inhibitor (PGSI)

drugs and birth control pills are the most effective ways to relieve menstrual cramps and long-standing pelvic pain.

4. Limitations from drugs used to treat menstrual cramps may include unpleasant side effects, which vary greatly from person to person.
5. The premenstrual syndrome is an aggregate of dozens of symptoms, resulting from female hormonal changes before menstruation. Treatment usually attempts to relieve the most common or incapacitating symptoms.
6. Chronic pelvic pain is usually unrelated to the menstrual cycle. It can be caused by a variety of problems, such as endometriosis, scar tissue, tumors, or infection of any of the female organs or of the nearby bowel or bladder. If painkillers, antibiotics, and hormone pills do not work, surgery may be necessary to treat these problems.
7. Pelvic pain is perhaps the major reason for the doctor to perform a diagnostic laparoscopy procedure. Laparoscopy and a D&C are safe, quick operations that are done while the woman is under general anesthesia. Unless there are extenuating medical reasons, removing the uterus or ovaries or cutting the nerve that transmits pelvic pain is not justified in treating pelvic pain.
8. Even if you become discouraged because your pelvic pain does not disappear after certain kinds of treatment have been initiated, continue to work with your physician toward exploring the cause and finding effective forms of treatment. Be sure to discuss openly any problems you have with alcoholism, stress, marital discord, or sexual difficulties.

11 Fertility Drugs

Unless they wish to have very large families, most women and their partners spend a large proportion of their reproductive years attempting to control their fertility. A significant minority of couples have the opposite problem, however, and their lives are often focussed on attempts to conceive and bear a child. Their problem is called infertility, and it affects about 10% of all couples who want to become parents. Worrying about unwanted pregnancies—and having them—is certainly painful, but the agonies of people who want to have babies and cannot may go even deeper. Years of frustration and dashed hopes may go by, with endless experimentation. Trips are made to different clinics and doctors, often very far from home; uncomfortable, painful, and even risky surgical procedures are undertaken; and rituals from the annals of folk medicine are tried, all to no avail. Besides the frustration of not getting results, unproductive attempts to solve infertility can put emotional, sexual, and financial strain on a couple's relationship.

Causes of infertility

The medical definition of infertility is the inability to conceive after a year of frequent intercourse without using contraceptive protection of any sort. If a couple continues for at least a year without success, they may consult an obstetrician-gynecologist who specializes in infertility problems. It is highly important that both the man and the woman cooperate in solving infertility problems. Regardless of the source of the problem, both partners will have to act in close cooperation with the physician when the attempt to conceive begins.

About 50% of the infertility cases brought to the attention of physicians concern problems with the woman's reproductive system; at least 40% are due to problems with the man's reproductive system. In about 10% of the cases the cause of infertility is due either to a combined problem of both the man and the woman or to causes that simply cannot be determined. Of the 50% that represents the female proportion of infertility, about 5% concern a problem with cervical mucus; about 30% are due to an obstruction of the fallopian tubes or a problem with the ovaries, the cervix or the uterus; and about 15% are due to lack of ovulation (egg production). Cervical mucus problems may be treated with antibiotics if there is an infection or with estrogen if the mucus is too thick. Surgery will sometimes help a blocked fallopian tube, but often the infertility continues after the unblocking because related problems still exist. There are procedures available to help with problems such as a cervix that is not tight enough to hold a developing fetus. If conception takes place, the cervix can be tightened with stitches for the duration of the pregnancy. Problems such as endometriosis can be treated by surgery or hormone-suppressing drugs (Chapter 10). The most progress in conquering infertility has been made in the area of stimulation of egg production. Of the proportion of women who are infertile because they do not produce eggs, up to 25% can be made to produce an egg and subsequently to conceive.

The most common cause of infertility in men, and one that is easily correctable, is a condition called a varicocele, which is an enlarged vein in the spermatic cord near each testicle, much like the varicose veins people have in their legs. One study established that these varicoceles were the cause of about 40% of all male infertility. These can be corrected by a simple, surgical procedure that is sometimes done on an outpatient basis. The doctor simply ties off the enlarged vein and reroutes the blood through another vessel. Depending on how low the sperm counts were before operation, the operation is from 30% to 70% effective. Hormone supplements following the operation can improve these statistics greatly.

Good progress is being made currently on the other causes of male infertility such as glandular disorders and congenital defects of the reproductive organs.

What happens at the first office visit

Much of a couple's first visit to a gynecologist who specializes in infertility will involve a discussion and questioning on many aspects of the couple's lives. The doctor will need to know both of their medical histories, including any problems with their reproductive systems, their occupations, sports and recreational activities, and their sexual habits and techniques. The physician will attempt to explain the various causes of infertility and to dispel any fears and misinformation the couple may have. The doctor will then schedule a complete physical examination for both the man and the woman. After that a series of tests will be given to determine the cause of infertility.

Testing

The major tests given at the beginning of the infertility consultation are included in the following discussions. After the tests have been completed, the doctor will make recommendations on the treatment of the infertility problem. These recommendations may include a surgical procedure for either the man or the woman, medical treatment for the woman, a change of certain sexual or work habits, or, a fertility drug if it is clear that no egg is being produced.

Semen analysis

The man will have to provide a fresh tube of semen so that the number of sperm can be counted, their structure and movement analyzed, and the volume of the ejaculate (material in which the sperm move) measured.

Determination of egg production

The woman's basal body temperature will have to be measured during the monthly menstrual cycle. At the time of egg production the temperature goes up 0.5 to 1 degree F; when this occurs, the fact that she has produced an egg can be verified.

X-ray examination of uterus and fallopian tubes

A special x-ray examination, called a hysterosalpingogram, will be made. This consists of inserting radiopaque dye in the uterus through the cervix. Using the x-ray apparatus the doctor will watch the dye, checking primarily to see if there are any deformities of the uterine cavity and if the dye passes through the fallopian tubes and spills out. If it does not, fallopian tube blockage is indicated.

Postcoital cervical mucus test

This test must be performed around the time of ovulation, which usually occurs 2 weeks before the onset of menstruation. The couple will be asked to have intercourse 2 to 4 hours before the test is made. The doctor will then examine the mucus that surrounds the cervix. Normal cervical mucus at the time of ovulation should be stringy, thin, and clear (this is known as *spinnbarkheit* mucus). Under a microscope the action of the sperm in the mucus is examined, and then a sperm count is done. It is desirable to see more than five sperm per high-power field through the microscope.

Stimulating egg production

The three most popular fertility drugs are clomiphene citrate (Clomid), a commercially prepared follicle-stimulating hormone and luteinizing hormone (Pergonal), and bromocriptine. Since each of these drugs acts in a different way, they are discussed separately.

Clomid

Clomid acts on two important brain centers, the pituitary gland and the hypothalamus, to stimulate production of the hormones that cause ovulation. Clomid counteracts the production of estrogen and thus induces the hypothalamus to produce luteinizing hormone and follicle-stimulating hormone. These are the hormones that actually cause the egg to ripen and be released. If anovulation (lack of egg release) is caused by severe pituitary gland or hypothalamus dysfunction, Clomid will probably not work.

Dosage schedule. In the Clomid treatment cycle, 5 days after the start of menstruation (which is often artificially induced) the woman receives 50 mg of Clomid in tablet form daily for 5 days. She stops the Clomid at that point, and ovulation should occur from 5 to 11 days later. Ovulation must be monitored closely, and intercourse will have to be carefully timed to correspond with its occurrence. If the Clomid cycle does not work, the daily dosage can be increased 50 mg each time it is tried (up to 250 mg per day). The treatment is sometimes prolonged by 2 more days. However, both prolonged treatment and higher dosages can result in overstimulation of the ovary and the production of more than one egg.

If fertilization has not occurred after three to six treatment cycles with Clomid, retesting for other problems must begin. Sperm counts, fallopian tube opening, conditions of the uterus, and quality of the cervical mucus should all be examined. Usually, fertilization will take place within the first three cycles. If after six cycles pregnancy has not yet occurred, the likelihood of it happening, at least by means of Clomid therapy, is small, and there is no point in continuing the drug.

Adverse effects. The most highly publicized problem with fertility drugs is multiple births. Sometimes the media give the impression that taking fertility pills guarantees quintuplets. However, the incidence of women taking Clomid and producing more than two children is less than 1%. The incidence of twins is 4% to 9%, with almost all of these being fraternal (nonidentical) twins. Multiple births result from excessive stimulation (hyperstimulation) of the ovaries, which can also create temporary ovarian enlargement, another undesirable side effect of Clomid. Ovarian enlargement probably occurs in fewer than 10% of women taking Clomid, although some studies have reported this figure to be as high as 13%. When ovarian enlargement does occur, Clomid treatments should be suspended until the problem can be more fully assessed.

The other major problem for women taking fertility drugs is the increased rate of spontaneous abortion, that is, miscarriage. For women who have taken Clomid the rate of miscarriage is 20%, whereas in normal conceptions it is 10% to 12%. When a woman has tried for years to become pregnant and finally succeeds in doing so only to lose her child through miscarriage, it can be a harsh blow. Once it has been established, however, that she can conceive using Clomid, she should take heart and try again, if her physician sees no contraindications to her making another attempt.

The number of birth defects reported for women who take

Clomid is no higher than those found in women who were treated for infertility in other ways. A slightly higher incidence of birth defects has been reported when women accidentally took Clomid after becoming pregnant (5.1% versus 2% to 4% in the normal population).

Pergonal

Whereas Clomid stimulates the production of the hormones necessary to induce ovulation, Pergonal is actually composed of those hormones. Use of Pergonal is indicated when treatment with Clomid has not worked, probably because pituitary and hypothalamus function are so poor that even strong stimulation couldn't cause them to produce the ovary-stimulating hormones. Pergonal is a 1:1 compound of luteinizing hormone and follicle-stimulating hormone extracted from the urine of menopausal women. Although the idea of merely supplying the needed hormones seems simpler than trying to make the body produce them, it is actually more difficult. Pergonal is more expensive than Clomid, it must be given intramuscularly, it requires much closer monitoring by the doctor, and it has more severe side effects. Therefore we recommend that Pergonal be used only after Clomid or other appropriate drugs have failed to solve the infertility problem.

Dosage schedule. In a characteristic treatment cycle the woman receives a daily injection of Pergonal for 3 to 4 days. Concurrently she must keep a daily temperature chart, perform a daily examination of her cervical mucus and ovaries, and have a daily blood test to determine estrogen levels. If the estrogen in her blood serum goes up, the same dosage of Pergonal should be continued. If it does not, the dosage should be increased for 3 more days. Twenty-four to 36 hours after the estrogen has reached a satisfactory level, an injection of another hormone, HCG (human chorionic gonadotropin), is given to maintain conception if it has taken place. If the estrogen levels have gone too high, the doctor will withhold the HCG shot, since high estrogen levels may indicate multiple egg production or ovarian enlargement. Four to 8 days later this hormone is reinjected to support the pregnancy if it has occurred. The incidence of pregnancy using this method is about 50%.

Adverse effects. Multiple births average about 25% when

this method of conquering infertility is used. Most of these are twins if the physician has been very cautious in monitoring the estrogen levels during the treatment cycle.

Ovarian hyperstimulation does occur in this program, but again careful monitoring of estrogen levels and withholding the HCG injection if they are too high should prevent the problem. A woman may have to be hospitalized if ovarian hyperstimulation occurs. In rare cases surgery will be necessary, for example, if an ectopic pregnancy (pregnancy outside the uterus) has occurred or the ovary is about to hemorrhage.

Miscarriage rates using Pergonal range from 20% to 25%; a significant portion of these miscarriages are two or more conceptions.

Bromocriptine

In a few cases of infertility the lack of ovulation is associated with excessive production by the body of prolactin, the hormone that stimulates the production of breast milk. Nursing mothers have high blood prolactin levels and are usually not as fertile as the normal population. In fact, many women never ovulate while they are nursing. Perhaps this is nature's way of helping women to space the births of their children. For some unknown reason the mechanism occasionally goes awry, and even though no baby has been born, the body produces prolactin.

The cause of the excessive prolactin production must be sought before bromocriptine is prescribed because tumors of the pituitary gland may be responsible. Since these tumors sometimes grow very rapidly during pregnancy, inducing conception may be dangerous when they are present.

Bromocriptine is taken in tablet form at bedtime because it may lower the blood pressure. The drug is taken every day for 4 weeks; if at the end of 4 weeks pregnancy has not resulted, the dosage is increased. Once again, ovulation must be monitored by temperature charts and, if it seems to occur, the drug should be stopped until menstruation begins.

The conception rate with bromocriptine used under these circumstances is at least 60%, and the number of miscarriages and birth defects associated with the use of this drug is thought to be the same as occurs in the normal population. When bromocriptine is first begun, women often experience nausea, headaches, low blood pressure, dizziness, and vomiting. These symptoms clear up with dosage adjustments and time.

Test tube babies

Research and scientific work in the area of infertility have made great progress over the past 10 years, particularly in the area of induction of ovulation, that is, causing a woman to produce an egg when she wasn't able to before. We estimate that, through various means, almost half of all infertile couples can create a pregnancy, and the majority of these will result in a healthy, normal child.

Test tube babies—babies produced by a process called in vitro fertilization—have fascinated the public recently. The first "test tube baby," a girl born on July 25, 1978, in England, now has dozens of counterparts that have been conceived in several other parts of the world.

How is a test tube baby created? The mother receives a drug like clomiphene (Clomid) or menotropins (Pergonal) to make her produce an egg, and preferably more than one egg at a predictable time. At just the right time, the eggs are suctioned out of a small incision in the abdomen through a long, telescope-like tube—the laparoscope. Next, the egg or eggs are incubated in a warm, moist chamber with a high carbon dioxide content, like that of the interior of the human body, for 6 to 8 hours. The father then contributes some fresh sperm, and the eggs and sperm are mixed carefully in a clear plastic dish.

For the next 2 days the doctors observe the contents of the dish, and when a four- to six-cell conception has been achieved, it is removed and inserted through the vagina into the mother's womb. If more than one conception has occurred, all are inserted. The most difficult hurdle comes next, that is, actual implantation in the wall of the uterus. As in nature, only about one in every four conceptions will successfully implant and go on to develop into a baby.

Chances are high that the entire process will have to be repeated, which is not only discouraging but also expensive, close to $5000 per attempt. Nevertheless, many couples go on to try again because the accomplishment of a pregnancy is the uppermost priority in their lives.

Personal experience

Brian and Cindi H had been married for 5 years, and during that time they had developed successful careers as a metallurgical engineer and an accountant, respectively. Cindi was fast approaching 30 when she and Brian agreed to put her diaphragm in the rear of the medicine cabinet so they could begin to start a family.

After over a year of regular, unprotected sexual activity and no sign of pregnancy, the couple suspected something was wrong. Cindi consulted her gynecologist, who examined both Brian and Cindi. Each was in good physical condition, with no obvious anatomical defects. Brian's sperm count was a healthy 40 million per milliliter and his sperm were vigorous and active. Cindi was then asked to take her temperature daily for a month. A clue appeared when her temperature never fluctuated more than two tenths of a degree, even when she would have presumably been ovulating. After obtaining the same temperature pattern for 3 consecutive months, Cindi's doctor decided that she was not ovulating.

Cindi began taking Clomid each day for the first 5 days following her menstrual period. As Cindi neared the fourteenth day of her cycle, her Clomid dosage was increased from 50 mg per day to 150 mg per day. At the same time she and Brian were told to plan intercourse for every other night from the tenth to the twentieth day of Cindi's menstrual cycle.

Three months went by and Cindi had still not become pregnant. The couple felt slightly discouraged and unhappy about the scheduled sex life necessary when using a fertility drug. Cindi's doctor told them to try 1 more month of Clomid, and if nothing happened she would prescribe another drug. At the end of the fourth month Cindi's menstrual period did not appear and she noticed some breast tenderness. A sensitive blood test showed up positive for pregnancy. Her doctor examined her by ultrasound 3 weeks later. The ultrasound image depicted a gestational sac and fetus about 8 weeks' size.

After an uncomplicated prenatal course Cindi went into labor near her estimated due date. Because the baby was in a breech position, the doctors decided to perform a cesarean. At that time they noted that Cindi's uterus, ovaries, and fallopian tubes appeared to be perfectly normal. She gave birth to a tiny but healthy 5-pound 8-ounce girl to the delight of her husband and the new grandparents.

THINGS TO REMEMBER

1. Infertility is a concern for about 10% of couples who wish to be parents. In approximately half of these couples the problems are due to a defect or deficiency of the female reproductive system.
2. Overcoming infertility takes a strong commitment to doing exactly what is necessary in the treatment cycle, and both partners must be equally committed to making it work, regardless of the source of the problem.
3. A careful history and physical examination of both the man and the woman must be obtained and a special regimen of tests conducted before a doctor can consider treating the infertility problem.
4. Clomid and Pergonal are the two major drugs used to treat infertility caused by lack of egg production occurring in approximately one third of women found to be infertile. Clomid is less expensive and has fewer side effects, so it is the first choice when the treatment cycle begins.
5. In special cases where lack of egg production is caused by excessive prolactin production, the drug bromocriptine has proved to be quite effective.
6. Very careful surveillance by both the patient and doctor are necessary to determine when ovulation occurs. The use of these fertility pills requires strict timing and patience if treatment fails.
7. The risk of miscarriage, birth defects, or twins with the use of fertility pills is low.
8. If a 3-month to 1-year trial of these medicines is unsuccessful, a reevaluation for other causes of infertility is indicated, and this may require diagnostic surgery. Ultimately the adoption of a child may be necessary.

12 Over-The-Counter Products for Women

Vaginal contraceptives

Today a woman can walk into a supermarket, discount department store, drugstore, or family planning clinic and purchase a large array of contraceptive items over the counter. She can choose from jellies, creams, aerosol foams, tablets, suppositories, and even tiny sponges. She need never consult a doctor, a pharmacist, or any health professional, yet she is still able to protect herself from unwanted pregnancy, provided that she knows what is in these products, how they work, and what their limitations are.

Statistics show that 80% of women who have intercourse without any contraceptive protection will become pregnant within a year. Unwanted pregnancies are an all too frequent occurrence. The most recent figures on the annual rate of legal induced abortion in the United States stand at 1,157,776 per year.* This figure represents one out of every 43 women in the reproductive age group (15 to 44) in the United States. A trip to the pharmacy to purchase a discreetly packaged purse-size contraceptive is well worth a woman's time if there is any chance that she will be sexually active.

Only one egg and one sperm are needed to produce a conception, but in any given act of intercourse 60 million or more sperm are ejaculated into the female reproductive tract and are at least potentially available to fertilize the one egg produced by the fe-

*Centers for Disease Control: Abortion Surveillance, 1978, US/DHS Bureau of Epidemiology, Family Planning Evaluation Division, Atlanta, Ga.

male. A variety of methods can prevent this. Effective contraception stops all of these sperm from uniting with the egg (fertilization). With over-the-counter products contraception usually immobilizes the sperm after they have entered the vagina or mechanically prevents them from entering the cervix (opening to the uterus) or the lower womb. These chemical vaginal contraceptives are called spermicides (sperm killers) because they prevent sperm from moving and cause them to die soon afterward. Having the spermicidal material spread over the mouth of the cervix also establishes a barrier through which the sperm simply cannot move.

Various compounds are used to immobilize and kill sperm, but probably the most common one found in over-the-counter materials is nonoxynol 9, a detergent that causes the outer cell membranes of the sperm to dissolve, thus preventing the sperm from moving. Nonoxynol 9 is the most common substance of its kind used for spermicidal contraceptives.

Four types of preparations of chemical vaginal contraceptives are currently on the market: the creams, jellies, or pastes usually squeezed from a tube; suppositories; gels; and foams, found in tablet form or in pressurized containers. Chemical vaginal contraceptives are inexpensive, easy to obtain, usually harmless, and somewhat effective.

The type of vaginal contraceptive chosen depends on personal preferences. Some women like creams because they provide extra lubrication in the vagina. Jellies are water soluble and easy to wash away. Certain creams and jellies are manufactured specially for use with a diaphragm; the diaphragm itself must be obtained by prescription. The combination of the diaphragm with a cream or jelly has long been considered a highly reliable and safe form of contraception because it combines a spermicide and two barriers. Physicians recommend this form of contraception rather than the use of a spermicide alone because it is much more dependable. Theoretically diaphragm use with spermicide is about 96% to 98% effective, but figures on actual use indicate it prevents pregnancy about 83% of the time.

Most physicians believe that contraceptive failures are caused in large part by incorrect or inconsistent usage. Jellies and creams meant to be used by themselves have a chemical composition and consistency different from those designed to team up with a diaphragm. They sometimes contain substances to make the pH (acid versus alkaline balance) of the vagina very acidic, an environment in which sperm cannot live. A woman inserts this type of jelly or cream with an applicator that contains the contraceptive material and a plunger to push it into the vagina. Buyers should read the labels carefully to determine which type of cream or jelly they are purchasing. They also need to carefully follow package directions on how long to wait to have intercourse after inserting the contraceptive material and how long to leave it undisturbed in place after having intercourse. With creams and jellies, either with or without a diaphragm, this is usually 8 or 9 hours after intercourse. After this time, if she wishes to, a woman may douche safely.

Foams and suppositories are conveniently packaged, easy to carry, and just as easy to insert. Both are placed deep in the vagina with an applicator or plunger device similar to that used for creams and jellies. Some women feel they cannot be detected during use, and that they leak very little after intercourse. Foaming tablets and suppositories should be inserted within 10 to 20 minutes before having intercourse. This gives them time to disintegrate and react with the body temperature and fluids to form the proper consistency for effective contraceptive action. None of the vaginal contraceptives should be inserted longer than an hour before intercourse takes place. Also, in every case a woman must put in a fresh application of contraceptive material before she has intercourse again. She should wait at least 8 or 9 hours after intercourse has taken place before douching or rinsing away the contraceptive foam.

On paper, foams and suppositories are up to 97% reliable. In actual practice the number looks more like 78% to 85%. We do not believe this number is high enough to recommend foams or suppositories alone for trustworthy contraception.

"Natural" sponges from oceanic origins have been advertised recently, appealing to those who do not want "unnatural" or chemical substances in their bodies. These sponges are designed to cover the cervical opening. Not enough information is available to evaluate the sponges in a fair way, but combined with a cream, jelly, or other type of spermicide they may be effective, provided they are inserted very carefully.

Some of our mothers used douching as a method of birth control. This may explain why so many of us came from families containing several children. Currently, douching is not recommended as a form of contraception. Sperm can reach the cervix as rapidly as 90 seconds from the time they enter the vagina, and 5 minutes later they can be in the fallopian tubes, where conception takes place. Most women are not able to nor would they probably care to douche that quickly. Nor can douching be considered thorough enough to rinse the millions of sperm from the vaginal tract. Douching must be avoided for at least 9 hours after intercourse when a vaginal spermicide is used, since douching will dilute the spermicide and render the mechanical barrier less effective.

The only truly effective vaginal contraceptives are those which are used in combination with a diaphragm or a condom. We do not recommend the use of spermicides by themselves because their reliability is not high enough, although they are better than no protection at all.

Vaginal spermicides are usually nontoxic. Occasionally they will irritate the vagina, the labia, or the penis. Some people report a sensation of heat or burning with effervescent suppositories like Encare. If this happens, use of the particular product causing the irritation should be stopped and a new product with different ingredients substituted. Chances are that a fragrance or another additive caused the problem rather than the active spermicidal ingredients. Although the spermicide is a poisonous substance, the dose in a vaginal contraceptive is so low that it probably would not be dangerous even if eaten.

Early in 1982 a report in the *Journal of the American Medical Association* stated that, among a large group of women studied, more children with congenital birth defects were born to those who had been using a vaginal spermicide around the time of conception than to those who had used no spermicide. The idea that spermicides are harmful to unborn babies is new, and there hasn't been enough time for researchers to evaluate it thoroughly. At this point we would not recommend terminating a pregnancy because a vaginal contraceptive had been used at the time of conception or in early pregnancy. However, it is advisable, if you are planning to become pregnant, to discontinue the use of vaginal spermicides at least 1 month before you begin your attempts.

Table 12-1 lists the most popular vaginal contraceptive products on the market today according to type. Table 12-2 gives the comparative effectiveness of various well-known contraceptive techniques.

Table 12-1 Vaginal contraceptives and their manufacturers

Creams
- Conceptrol (Ortho)
- Delfen (Ortho)

Gels/creams (to be used with diaphragm)
- Koromex II (cream) (Holland-Rantos)
- Koromex II (gel) (Holland-Rantos)
- Ortho-Creme (Ortho)
- Ortho-Gynol (Ortho)

Gels
- Koromex A II (Holland-Rantos)
- Ramses 10-Hour (Schmid)

Foams
- Because Birth Control Foam (Schering)
- Dalkon (Robins)
- Delfen (Ortho)
- Emko; Emko Pre-fil (Schering)
- Koromex (Holland-Rantos)

Suppositories
- Encare (Eaton-Merz)
- Intercept (Ortho)
- Semicid (Whitehall)
- S'Positive (Jordan-Simner)

Sponges
- Today (VLI)

Table 12-2 Comparative effectiveness of birth control methods

Method	Effective theoretical use (%)	Effective actual use (%) (U.S. women not wanting more children)
Abortion	100	100
Tubal ligation	99.96	99.96
Vasectomy	85 to 99	85 to 99
Combined oral contraceptive	99.66	90 to 96
Condom plus spermicide	99	95
IUD	97 to 99	95
Condom	97	90
Diaphragm plus spermicide	97	83
Spermicide	97	78
Coitus interruptus	91	75 to 80
Rhythm (calendar)	87	79
Lactation for 12 months	75	60
Chance (sexually active)	10	10

From Hatcher, R.A., et al.: Contraceptive technology, 1978-79, ed. 9, 1978. Reprinted with permission of Irvington Publishers, Inc., New York.

Home pregnancy tests

Recent advertisements in women's magazines are a revealing indicator of the popularity of the early pregnancy tests (EPTs). These tests allow a woman to diagnose pregnancy in the privacy of her home. They employ simple methods with a high rate of accuracy. The tests use dried red blood cells from sheep that react with a hormone in the urine of pregnant women—human chorionic gonadotropin (HCG). The test must be performed carefully, with the urine and cells left undisturbed in a dark place for 2 full hours after they have been shaken together. A doughnut-shaped circle will appear at the end of 2 hours if there is a pregnancy. Accuracy is about 97% for positive readings and 80% for negative readings. The manufacturers recommend that the test be repeated a week later if the user obtained a negative reading and still did not have her menstrual period. In the case of actual pregnancy, a false negative result is usually the result of the test being done too early. It is not sensitive until 9 or more days after the first period has been missed.

Early pregnancy tests may provide strong evidence that a pregnancy exists, but they are not a substitute for an early visit to the doctor. Ectopic pregnancy (pregnancy outside the uterus), for example, will produce negative results yet is a dangerous situation needing immediate medical attention. If a woman continues to suspect pregnancy, she should not hesitate to call her doctor, even if her EPT was negative, or to repeat the test in a week.

EPTs cost between $8 and $9 per kit and can be used only once. Family planning clinics such as Planned Parenthood will do pregnancy tests for about half that cost. The privacy of doing the test at home may outweigh the added costs for many people, which is fine as long as the test does not take the place of professional medical care.

Menstrual discomfort aids

Women experience a wide range of uncomfortable symptoms during their menstrual periods, even though menstruation is a normal function and ideally poses no more than minor inconveniences for a few days a month. Women with serious pain or swelling during menstruation need to seek the advice of a gynecologist. In recent years medical research has uncovered new information about the cause of menstrual discomfort. Physicians had long attributed the excessive cramps of menstruation to estrogenic hormones. Now they know that neurohormones called prostaglandins, formed by the endometrium (uterine lining), provoke the uterine contractions and pain of menstrual cramps. Because prostaglandins work their way into other body systems by way of the bloodstream, they may also cause diarrhea, nausea, and vomiting. Besides the discomfort caused by natural prostaglandins, diseases of the uterus such as tumors, cysts, polyps, or endometriosis may also cause painful menstruation. Conditions such as these tend to produce discomfort that comes on suddenly or gradually worsens, as compared with the menstrual pain caused by prostaglandins, which begins in adolescence.

A variety of over-the-counter products relieve these symptoms, which include headaches, fluid accumulation, backaches, breast tenderness, abdominal cramping, and irritability, anxiety, and depression. At least 15 preparations for relief of menstrual symptoms can be purchased over the counter (Table 12-3). Only a few basic ingredients make up these many different products. Most menstrual discomfort relief pills contain two or more of the following: (1) an analgesic, that is, a pain reliever such as aspirin or acetaminophen; (2) an antihistamine, which in menstrual products makes the user drowsy and perhaps less tense and nervous; (3) a diuretic (to get rid of excess fluid) such as caffeine, ammonium chloride, or pamabrom, which stimulate urination and decrease fluid retention; and (4) an antispasmodic such as ephedrine, which may help relieve cramping.

Only the analgesics, aspirin and acetaminophen, have any proved benefits for relief of menstrual symptoms. They relieve pain by actually blocking prostaglandin production. When you consider that the cost of menstrual products is substantially higher than plain aspirin or acetaminophen (and the value is nearly the same), you may wish to consider switching products. If these do not work, then specific drugs to block prostaglandins can be helpful. Some of these new drugs (Motrin, Ponstel, Anaprox) require a prescription.

The levels of an antihistamine or diuretic in most over-the-counter menstrual discomfort products are not high enough to effectively manage the problems they should correct. Women who have a lot of water retention before their periods will prob-

Table 12-3 Over-the-counter menstrual discomfort aids

Product and manufacturer	Ingredients
Aqua-Ban (Thompson Medical)	Ammonium chloride, 325 mg; caffeine, 100 mg
Cardui (Chattem)	Acetaminophen, 325 mg; pamabrom, 25 mg; pyrilamine maleate, 12.5 mg
Femcaps (Buffington)	Aspirin, 162 mg; phenacetin, 65 mg; caffeine, 32 mg; ephedrine sulfate 8 mg; atropine sulfate, 0.0325 mg
Midol (Glenbrook)	Aspirin, 454 mg; caffeine, 32.4 mg; cinnamedrine, 14.9 mg
Odrinil (water pills) (Fox)	Powdered extract of buchu, 34.4 mg; uva ursi, 34.4 mg; corn silk, 34.4 mg; juniper, 16.2 mg; caffeine extract, 16.2 mg
Pamprin (Chattem)	Acetaminophen, 325 mg; pamabrom, 25 mg; pyrilamine maleate, 12.5 mg
Permathene H_2Off (Alleghany)	Ammonium chloride, 600 mg; caffeine, 200 mg
Sunril Premenstrual Capsules (Schering)	Acetaminophen, 300 mg; pamabrom, 50 mg; pyrilamine maleate, 25 mg
Trendar Premenstrual Tablets (Whitehall)	Acetaminophen, 325 mg; pamabrom, 25 mg
Tri-Aqua (Pfeiffer)	Extracts of buchu, uva ursi, triticum, zea, and caffeine, 100 mg

ably benefit as much by restricting their salt intake at that time as by consuming pills. If you are very uncomfortable and your weight gain exceeds 4 pounds over normal before your period, consult your gynecologist for suggestions.

In summary, over-the-counter menstrual discomfort aids do provide relief for some women, but often their ingredients are not contained in sufficiently high quantities to really get the job done. They are safe, non-habit-forming, and not particularly expensive, although plain aspirin and acetaminophen are cheaper. Women who do not get adequate relief through these products should see a gynecologist. Many effective prescription drugs are available, some of them quite new, that block the production of prostaglandin and offer effective relief from menstrual discomfort. Today there is no longer a reason for women of any age to suffer from unrelenting cramps.

Tampons and sanitary napkins

Until 1979 the use of tampons versus sanitary napkins did not elicit much controversy. Then tampons were implicated in a serious, and in rare instances fatal, disease called toxic shock syndrome. Toxic shock syndrome is characterized by fever, very low blood pressure causing dizziness or faintness, a red skin rash, particularly on the hands and soles of the feet, vomiting, diarrhea, and severe muscle pain. Studies revealed that 98% of the cases of toxic shock syndrome reported were in menstruating women and appeared within 5 days of the start of a menstrual period. The Centers for Disease Control in Atlanta studied several hundred women who had suffered from toxic shock syndrome and found that the use of certain brands of highly absorbant tampons correlated with incidences of toxic shock syndrome. Staphylococcal bacteria in the vaginal tract were the infecting organisms.

Women deserted their favorite tampons in droves, and companies that manufactured tampons mobilized millions of dollars, not only for legal defense but also for research into the causes of toxic shock syndrome. Several brands of tampons were withdrawn from supermarket and drugstore shelves.

At this time researchers believe that tampons are not the sole cause of toxic shock syndrome (it has occurred in men and nonmenstruating women) but that there is a strong connection between the two, especially with the superabsorbant tampons. A tiny, symptom-free abrasion (scratch or sore spot) in the vagina, possibly caused by a tampon, often occurs with toxic shock, and a bacterial and pH imbalance in the vagina seems to be responsible for the excessive growth of the particular staphylococcal bacteria in question. The organisms are present either in the vagina itself or on the labia and are introduced somehow into the vaginal canal, possibly by a woman's own hands. If a woman notices any of the symptoms just described while she is wearing a tampon, she should remove the tampon immediately and seek medical attention.

Should a woman still use tampons? Knowing the facts, she should feel free to make the right choice for herself. Most of the highly absorbant tampons have been removed from stores and are not currently available. The less absorbant kind are probably safer although something of a nuisance because they may have to be combined with sanitary napkin use during times of heavy flow. Napkins themselves seem to be the safest choice, especially at night. They do need to be changed more often because they create more odor and menstrual fluid accumulation in the genital area. Some women complain of chafing and irritation from sanitary napkin use. If a woman does continue to use tampons, she should observe some simple rules:

1. Don't use superabsorbant tampons made with synthetic fibers. Use tampons made of cotton or mixtures of synthetics and cotton.
2. Change tampons at least once every 4 to 6 hours.
3. Use sanitary napkins at night while asleep.
4. Wash hands with soap and water before inserting a tampon.

Whatever she decides, a woman should be aware that the possibility of toxic shock syndrome during tampon use exists. However, the actual incidence of toxic shock syndrome in the menstruating population is extremely low, and the likelihood of contracting it is remote. We believe the press has overplayed the entire issue to a great degree.

Douches, sprays, and other feminine deodorant products

Certain social and cultural notions that a woman's genitalia are unclean and malodorous have become prevalent, especially in recent years. Women gradually took up the practices of douching, spraying, and applying directly various substances to sanitize their genital region.

Douches

The douche (the word origin is French) has been practiced for many decades. It originated in Europe, along with the bidet, a kind of built-in bathroom douching fixture. The principle of douching is to eject a jet of water, usually containing some sort of disinfectant or deodorizing material, into the vagina under pressure. Deodorant sprays, wipes, and other topical applications are relatively recent additions to drugstore and supermarket shelves.

The medical benefits of regular douching are controversial. A few studies have indicated that women who douche regularly have a healthier, stronger vaginal interior with a more favorable mix of the typical vaginal organisms. On the other hand, reports of women worsening vaginal infections by forcing organisms higher up into their reproductive tract have also appeared. Most gynecologists do not recommend the practice of douching, primarily because it doesn't do much good and can cause trouble.

Table 12-4 Feminine cleansing and deodorant products

Product and manufacturer	Ingredients
Betadine Douche (Purdue Frederick)	Povidone-iodine
Bo-Car-Al (Beecham)	Boric acid, phenol, menthol, methyl salicylate, eucalyptus oil, thymol, potassium aluminum sulfate
Demure (Vicks)	Benzethonium chloride, lactic acid
Femidine Douche (A.V.P.)	Povidone-iodine
Janeen (Norwich)	Lactic acid, sodium lactate, propylene glycol
Lysette (Lehn & Fink)	Triethanolamine dodecylbenzene sodium sulfonate, alcohol, 31%
Massengill Disposable Douche (Beecham)	Cetylpyridium chloride, alcohol, lactic acid, octoxynol, fragrance
Massengill Douche Powder (Beecham)	Boric acid, ammonium aluminum sulfate, berberine, fragrance
Massengill Liquid (Beecham)	Alcohol, lactic acid, sodium lactate, octoxynol, aromatics
Massengill Vinegar & Water Disposable Douche (Beecham)	Boric acid, vinegar
Nylmerate II (Holland-Rantos)	Boric acid, alcohol, 50%; acetic acid, polysorbate, 20%; nonoxynol-9, sodium acetate
PMC Douche Powder (Thomas & Thompson)	Boric acid, 82%; thymol, 0.3%; phenol, 0.2%; menthol, ammonium aluminum sulfate, 16%; eucalyptus oil, peppermint oil
Stomaseptine (Bertex)	Menthol, eucalyptol, and thymol, 2%; sodium perborate, 18%; sodium chloride, 28%; sodium borate, 25%; sodium bicarbonate, 25%
Trichotine Liquid and Powder (Reed Carnrick)	Sodium perborate, sodium borate, aromatics, sodium lauryl sulfate, alcohol, 8% (liquid)
V.A. (Norcliff Thayer)	Boric acid, 8-hydroxyquinoline citrate, zinc sulfate, alum
Zonite (Norcliff Thayer)	Benzalkonium chloride, menthol, thymol, propylene glycol, buffer

The most common complication of douching seems to be irritation of the labia and vagina. Simple vinegar or baking soda douches probably do not often create irritation, but some of the commercially manufactured douche products could easily do so. Benzalkonium, benzethonium chloride, chlorhexidine hydrochloride, and chloroxylenol are added as preservatives to counteract bacteria, not in the vagina but in the douching material. Phenol and benzocaine exert a local anesthetic effect and may help relieve the discomfort of vaginal itching. Ammonium and potassium alums and zinc sulfate are astringents, substances that cause skin or mucous membranes to contract or tighten up. Astringents may help to relieve swelling, inflammation, and exudation (drops of liquid leaking through the skin), but they can also be irritating and cause a rebound effect. When using a commercially prepared douche product, carefully read the label to see what the ingredients are. Table 12-4 lists popular douche and deodorant products and their ingredients and should prove helpful as an aid in selecting douches. If douching is necessary, we recommend a simple preparation of 1 tablespoon of white vinegar mixed with 1 quart of lukewarm water.

Aside from knowing what is in douche preparations and what they do, the most important consideration in douching is how to do it properly. Following are some guidelines:

1. Douche liquids should never be instilled with excess pressure. The force of gravity is usually sufficient. When using a hand-held syringe, minimum pressure should be exerted.
2. Most douches should be instilled while a woman is lying down in the bathtub with her knees drawn up and hips raised.
3. Water used to dilute douche preparations should be lukewarm, not hot.
4. Douching should be limited to no more than twice a week.
5. Douching should not be done during pregnancy.

Feminine deodorant products

Feminine deodorant sprays and premoistened towelettes have to be regarded as cosmetics and not medications. Their primary ingredient is perfume, and their purpose is to mask odors in the female genital region. Manufacturers claim that they are safe if correctly used, but many physicians have noted problems attributable to the use of these deodorant products, such as irritation and allergic sensitization. Perhaps, when used correctly, these materials are not harmful to the majority of women, but there is no way their use can be controlled in the general population.

If used, the sprays should be held at least 9 inches from the body and should not be sprayed directly on either the inner labia or in the vagina. They should not be used immediately after intercourse nor applied more than once a day. Most evidence indicates that washing daily with a mild soap and warm water achieves the same deodorizing effect as sprays or towelettes, with fewer side effects. Around the time of the menstrual period, changing pads and tampons frequently holds down odors for the vast majority of women.

Topical anesthetics and anti-itch products

Numerous over-the-counter products contain local anesthetics, antihistamines, astringents, antibacterial agents, and anti-irritants, including a cortisone cream for application to the skin (hydrocortisone). Until 1981 hydrocortisone was available only through prescription, but now it can be found in a number of commercially available products in rather low concentrations. Table 12-5 lists several of these products and the ingredients in them. They can provide welcome relief from some of the itching and irritation of vaginal infections or discomfort after the birth of a baby. On the other hand, they should not be used to replace medical treatment for underlying infections. Women should watch for signs of allergic reaction and stop using these medications if they occur. Most dermatologists recommend discriminating, careful use of hydrocortisone and advise against daily application for any prolonged period.

Table 12-5 Creams and lotions to relieve feminine itching and soreness

Product and manufacturer	Ingredients
Antihistamines	
Benadryl (Parke-Davis)	Diphenhydramine HCl, 2%; water-miscible base
PBZ (Geigy)	Tripelennamine HCl, 2% Cream: water-washable base Ointment: petrolatum base

Table 12-5 Creams and lotions to relieve feminine itching and soreness – cont'd

Product and manufacturer	Ingredients
Anesthetics	
Americaine (American Critical Care)	Benzocaine, 20% Aerosol: water-dispersible base Ointment: water-soluble polyethylene glycol base; benzethonium chloride, 0.1%
Benzocaine (various)	Benzocaine, 5%; cream, ointment base
Butesin Picrate (Abbott)	Butamben picrate, 1%; ointment base
Dibucaine (various)	Dibucaine, 1%; ointment base
Nupercainal (CIBA)	Dibucaine, 0.5%; water-washable base
Pontocaine (Breon)	Tetracaine HCl, 1%; water-miscible base
Quotane (Menley & James)	Dimethisoquin HCl, 0.5%; thimerosal 1:50,000; water-miscible base
Surfacaine (Lilly)	Cream: cyclomethycaine, 0.5%; vanishing cream base Ointment: cyclomethycaine sulfate, 1%
Tronothane (Abbott)	Pramoxine HCl, 1% Cream: water-miscible base Jelly: water-soluble base
Xylocaine (Astra)	Lidocaine, 2.5%; water-miscible base
Corticosteroids	
Clearaid (Squibb)	Hydrocortisone, 0.5%
Cortaid (Upjohn)	Hydrocortisone acetate equivalent to hydrocortisone, 0.5%; ointment, cream, or spray
Dermolate Anti-Itch (Schering)	Hydrocortisone, 0.5%; cream, spray
Combination products	
Aerotherm (Aeroceuticals)	Spray: benzocaine, 13.6%; benzyl alcohol, 22.7%
Bicozene Creme (Ex-Lax)	Benzocaine, 5%; resorcinol 1.67%
Derma-Medicone (Medicone)	Benzocaine, 2%; oxyquinoline sulfate, 1.05%; menthol, 0.28%; ichthammol, 1%; zinc oxide, 13.7%; petrolatum, lanolin, perfume
Dermoplast (Ayerst)	Spray: benzocaine, 20%; menthol, 0.5%; water-miscible base
Diothane (Merrell-National)	Diperodon, 1%; petrolatum; propylene glycol; sorbitan sesquioleate; oxyquinoline benzoate, 0.1%
Foille (Blistex)	Spray: benzocaine, 2%; benzyl alcohol, 4%; oxyquinoline; vegetable oil base
Pontocaine (Breon)	Tetracaine, 0.5%; menthol, 0.5%; white petrolatum, white wax
Tucks (Parke-Davis)	Premoistened pads: witch hazel, 50%; glycerin, 10%; water; methylparaben, 0.1%; benzethonium chloride, 0.003%
Vaginex (Schmid)	Benzocaine, resorcinol
Vagisil Feminine Itching Medication (Combe)	Benzocaine, 5%; resorcinol, 2%

Lubricants

Lubricants such as H-R Lubricating Jelly and K-Y Lubricating Jelly can be safely used for dryness in the vagina during intercourse. These products are inexpensive and harmless. If dryness continues, especially if a woman is undergoing menopause, estrogen replacement therapy may be prescribed by a physician.

Diet pills

Estimates of the number of people in the United States who are actually obese, that is, 20% above their ideal body weight, range between 25% and 35% of the entire population. The number of people who consider themselves fat and wish to be thinner goes somewhat beyond that. The majority of these are women. Furthermore, the stereotyped ideal of the American woman is a tall, willowy creature with most of her skeletal structure discernible through a thin layer of skin. Small wonder, then, that over-the-counter diet pills and preparations are big sellers. Some women struggle throughout their lives with weight loss, often as early as adolescence, using every manner at hand to reduce.

The most common substance found in over-the-counter diet pills is phenylpropanolamine, which is chemically related to the ephedrines and amphetamines. Several products also contain fairly high doses of caffeine. All these drugs have a strong stimulating effect on the body's nervous system, and women who take any of them often feel very energetic, even hyperactive, as well as less hungry. Although some controversy over the safety of phenylpropanolamine has been generated, an FDA (Food and Drug Administration) advisory panel recently approved it as safe and effective when used in the proper dosages for no more than 12 consecutive weeks. This recommended dosage was recently reduced from 150 mg per day to 75 mg per day.

Like amphetamines, phenylpropanolamine can cause unpleasant side effects, such as nervous anxiety, restlessness, insomnia, headache, nausea, and high blood pressure. These tend to occur when the normal recommended dosages have been exceeded. A dosage of 25 to 30 mg every 4 hours and no more than 75 mg in 24 hours is considered safe. Several of the leading brands of diet pills contain considerably higher doses than that. People with diabetes, heart disease, high blood pressure, or thyroid problems should consult with their doctors before taking phenylpropanolamine. Commonly available weight-reduction pills containing phenylpropanolamine are listed in Table 12-6 along with the dosages and other ingredients.

Certain drugs that produce calorie-free bulk, such as cellulose, are now sold for weight-reduction purposes. Some of the popular brands are listed in Table 12-6. Research indicates that bulk production does not really contribute to significant weight loss, since a bulky mass is almost entirely gone from the stomach in 30 minutes. Bulk-producing substances also have a laxative side effect, which may not always be desirable. Some of

Table 12-6 Over-the-counter diet pills and aids

Product and manufacturer	Phenylpropanolamine hydrochloride (mg)	Bulk producer	Other ingredients
Anorexin Capsules (SDA Pharmaceuticals)	25	Carboxymethylcellulose sodium, 50 mg	Caffeine, 100 mg; vitamin A, 1667 IU; vitamin D, 133 IU; thiamine, 1 mg; riboflavin, 1 mg; pyridoxine hydrochloride, 0.33 mg; cyanocobalamin, 0.33 gm; ascorbic acid, 20 mg; niacinamide, 7 mg; calcium pantothenate, 0.33 mg
Appedrine Tablets (Thompson)	25	Carboxymethylcellulose sodium, 50 mg	Caffeine, 100 mg; vitamin A, 1667 IU; vitamin D, 133 IU; thiamine, 1 mg; riboflavin, 1 mg; pyridoxine hydrochloride, 0.33 mg; cyanocobalamin, 0.33 gm; ascorbic acid, 20 mg; niacinamide, 7 mg; calcium pantothenate, 0.33 mg
Appress (North American)	25	–	Caffeine, 100 mg
Ayds Appetite Suppressant Droplets (Purex)	25	–	–
Coffee Break Cubes Weight Reduction Plan (O'Connor)	37.5	–	–
Coffee, Tea & a New Me (Thompson)	25	–	–

Continued.

Table 12-6 Over-the-counter diet pills and aids—cont'd

Product and manufacturer	Phenylpropanolamine hydrochloride (mg)	Bulk producer	Other ingredients
Dex-A-Diet II (O'Connor)	75	–	Caffeine, 200 mg
Dexatrim Capsules (Thompson)	50	–	Caffeine, 200 mg
Diadax Capsules (O'Connor)	50	–	–
Diadax Tablets (O'Connor)	25	–	–
Diet-Trim Tablets (Pharmex)	Not significant	Carboxymethylcellulose	Benzocaine
Grapefruit Diet Plan with Diadax Tablets (O'Connor)	10	–	Natural grapefruit extract, 16.6 mg; ascorbic acid, 10 mg; vitamin E, 3.6 mg
Grapefruit Diet Plan with Diadax Vitamin Fortified Continuous Action Capsules (O'Connor)	30	–	Natural grapefruit extract, 50 mg; ascorbic acid, 30 mg; vitamin E, 11 mg
Grapefruit Diet Plan with Diadax Chewable Tablets, Extra Strength (O'Connor)	25	–	Natural grapefruit extract, 33 mg; ascorbic acid, 20 mg; vitamin E, 10 IU
Grapefruit Diet Plan with Diadax Extra Strength Vitamin Fortified Continuous Action Capsules (O'Connor)	75	–	Natural grapefruit extract, 100 mg; ascorbic acid, 60 mg; vitamin E, 30 IU
Odrinex Tablets (Fox)	25	Methylcellulose, 50 mg	Caffeine, 50 mg
Pro-Dax 21 (O'Connor)	75	–	–
Prolamine Capsules (Thompson)	35	–	Caffeine, 140 mg
Slim-Line Candy (O'Connor)	–	Methylcellulose, 45 mg	Benzocaine, 5 mg; corn glucose syrup; natural and artificial flavoring
Slim-Line Gum (O'Connor)	–	–	Benzocaine, 6 mg
Spantrol Capsules (North American)	75	Carboxymethylcellulose sodium, 135 mg	Caffeine (anhydrous), 150 mg; benzocaine, 9 mg; ascorbic acid, 30 mg; thiamine hydrochloride, 1 mg; riboflavin, 1.2 mg; niacinamide, 10 mg; pyridoxine hydrochloride, 1 mg iron, 10 mg

the methylcellulose wafers can cause esophageal obstruction and should be consumed with plenty of water. A few drugs—anticholinergics—slow down bowel action and, when used with bulk producers, could create intestinal blockage. Obviously, the two should not be used together. Diphenoxylate (Lomotil), a prescription drug used for diarrhea control, is one example.

Benzocaine, a local anesthetic, is sometimes incorporated into weight-control preparations. It may numb the inside of the mouth slightly or, if swallowed, the lining of the bowel. Its weight-loss effects, if any, appear to be very subtle. There are reports of a few serious side effects with its use, such as shortness of breath and severe allergic reaction leading to death. Some people may become allergic to the drug after long-term use.

Other diet preparations available are low-calorie balanced foods, diet candies, and artificial sweeteners, all of which may or may not assist in weight loss, depending on the individual.

Pregnant women should not use diet preparations, particularly drugs containing phenylpropanolamine. Pregnancy is not the time to go on a weight-loss program. Women should concentrate on eating a nutritious well-balanced diet while they are expecting a baby, and often this is best achieved by eating four or five light meals per day. For pregnant women who are already overweight, the goal should not be to lose weight while pregnant, but to concentrate on weight loss after their babies are safely delivered.

Most people find that diet pills and preparations are but temporary measures to get them slimmer. Once they are discontinued, the pounds tend to inch back. Commitment to a nutritious but low-calorie diet and a suitable exercise program is much more effective. For most obese people this means a permanent change in life-style and attitude as well as eating and exercise habits. They have to decide if a slender and probably healthier body is sufficient reward for the effort.

■ Personal experience

Deloris F was married, with three youngsters ranging in ages from 7 to 12. She and her husband were happy with the size of their family and enjoying their lives more now that their children were older and less dependent. Deloris was in good health, except for the 20 extra pounds she had not lost since her last pregnancy. Finding it hard to stick to a diet, Deloris purchased Dexatrim at her local supermarket from time to time, hoping that the pills would suppress her appetite. She usually lost about 5 pounds and gained them back rapidly as soon as she discontinued the drug.

Now 35, Deloris smoked a pack of cigarettes a day. Because of this she was unable to take contraceptive pills. She had always been afraid to try an IUD because several of her friends had had bad experiences with it. Her periods had always been very regular, so she used the rhythm method and then Delfen foam for contraception. Deloris also liked to use Massengill Disposable Douche following intercourse as a deodorant and cleanser.

When she missed her usually regular period, she was taken by surprise. She and her husband purchased an EPT, and their experiment yielded positive results. Deloris told the doctor she couldn't understand what had happened because their contraceptive regimen had worked for 7 years. On close questioning the doctor learned that Deloris had douched only 3 hours after intercourse at a date midway through her menstrual cycle. Deloris was reminded that a woman should wait at least 8 hours before douching after intercourse. Although taken aback by this unplanned pregnancy, Deloris and her husband decided not to have an abortion. They are scheduling a genetic amniocentesis to be done at the end of her fourth month of pregnancy.

THINGS TO REMEMBER

1. Vaginal contraceptives are inexpensive and readily available, but we do not recommend their use alone. For truly reliable contraception, they should be used in combination with a barrier method like the diaphragm, condom, or sponge.
2. Early pregnancy tests help a woman determine for herself whether she is pregnant. They are more accurate when positive results are achieved. If the test is negative and menstruation still does not begin, repeat the test or visit your doctor.
3. Drugstore counters contain a variety of products to relieve menstrual distress. Even though they often contain several ingredients, the most effective are plain aspirin and acetaminophen.
4. The more serious forms of menstrual distress can be treated

with some new prescription drugs that have been developed over the past couple of years (see Chapter 10).

5. Use of certain superabsorbant tampons has been associated with toxic shock syndrome. If you notice any of the symptoms of toxic shock beginning to occur, remove any tampon you are wearing and quickly seek medical attention.
6. If you do wish to use tampons, buy the less absorbant ones made of cotton. Change tampons frequently, use sanitary napkins at night, and wash hands with soap and water before inserting a tampon.
7. Regular douching has little or no medical benefit. Occasionally a warm water douche with 1 tablespoon of white vinegar or baking soda will relieve itching or discomfort caused by a discharge.
8. If you want to douche, use warm but never hot water. Pressure from the force of gravity is high enough to push water into the vagina. Douche no more than twice a week, and never douche when pregnant.
9. Over-the-counter diet pills can provide short-term weight loss. They often have side effects, especially if the recommended dosages are exceeded, and once they are discontinued, weight tends to return.

13 Herpes and Other Genital Infections

The thought of contracting a sexually transmitted or venereal disease has always been appalling, but recently this particular anxiety reached mass proportions. The national consciousness riveted itself on venereal disease, particularly herpes, an ailment that became a household word. Magazines, newspapers, books, and television talk shows all examined in exquisite detail not only the symptoms of herpes, but also its psychological impact on sufferers. People who had been unfortunate enough to contract the disease began to band together, forming support groups and networks. Singles groups and dating services that matched up male and female herpes victims were established so that conscience-stricken herpes victims would not contaminate those who had not been exposed to the disease, but instead limit their sexual relationships to one another.

Yet virtually all women who have ever been sexually active have had infections that are sexually relevant, if not actually sexually transmitted. Most of these are treatable, and the rest are controllable. Our purpose in writing this chapter is to discuss the common genital infections and their treatment, and also to reassure women that they need not feel unclean or outcast because they have a genital infection, even if it is herpes. The important thing to remember if you suspect you have a genital infection is to visit your physician promptly and inform your sexual partners, so that they can have the benefit of treatment too, if necessary.

Infections of the labia and external genital organs most commonly present themselves as sores. Inflammations of the vagina, known as vaginitis, usually lead to itching or a foul-smelling discharge. More serious internal infections of the uterus, ovaries, and fallopian tubes can cause fever, pain, swelling, tenderness, nausea, and diarrhea. Not all sores or discharges are caused by infection, and this is a strong reason for getting medical help at the earliest possible moment. Particularly in women beyond menopause, these problems can signal cancer or a premalignancy situation.

The term *sexually transmitted* in reference to genital infections could probably be rephrased more accurately as sexually transmittable. Often these infections result from a woman engaging in sexual relations with someone who is already infected. In some cases, though, they may begin because a woman has taken antibiotics, douched with the wrong substance, or even used a contaminated toilet seat or dirty towel. Once these diseases are activated, however, they can be passed on to sexual partners, and thus they are accurately termed *venereal diseases.*

Genital sores

Most women we see in our clinics who have genital sores have nothing more remarkable than a skin abrasion, a blemish, or an infected hair follicle. If the sore is blistered or bleeding and craterlike, then we suspect something more serious like herpes or even cancer.

Herpes

The incidence of herpes infections in the United States is estimated to be between 15 and 20 million, and a half million new victims join this statistic each year. Men outnumber women in the ranks of herpes sufferers, and among both sexes most of these people are between the ages of 18 and 35. This epidemic is assumed to reflect the sexually liberal attitudes of the past 15 years, and it is probably also related to the post-World War II population boom in this same age group.

Two types of herpes viruses exist. The first, herpes type I, usually does not affect the reproductive organs, but instead causes cold sores around the lips. The other, herpes type II, appears on the genitals and is usually transmitted sexually. Although the two viruses are very closely related, the herpes type II strain is more worrisome. Not only does it tend to cause greater pain and discomfort, but also women who have herpes show a higher incidence of cervical cancer than those who have never contracted the infection.

Herpes can break out any time from 2 days to 2 weeks after contact with a carrier. The typical attack begins with a burning or itching sensation in the genital area followed by the appearance of small, slightly raised bumps. Blisters form and then rupture, leaving tiny ulcers or clusters of ulcers that weep fluid. Most herpes infections run their course between 3 and 6 weeks after breaking out if it is the primary, or first, infection. Secondary infections last about 7 to 14 days. They must be kept very clean and as dry as possible to prevent their contamination with bacteria; otherwise, a consequent bacterial infection could take over from the herpes viral one.

One of the most unfortunate aspects of the herpes virus is that, once contracted, it remains in the body to appear again and again over the years. After a herpes infection has healed, the virus ascends the nerves that lead to the genitals and hides within the nerve roots near the spine until something precipitates its reappearance. Scientists can only speculate on why herpes is able to keep itself alive like this, but one theory holds that the herpes mutates or changes just enough after each infection that the antibodies formed by the person with herpes cannot destroy it.

Although the first infection is usually the worst in terms of physical symptoms, it is probably the recurring outbreaks that create high levels of psychological distress in victims. Repeated outbreaks seem to have some causal relationship to stress and anxiety. Psychologists have identified a herpes-related syndrome in which people with the disease feel rejected by society, become very depressed, and withdraw from social contact. They recommend that people experiencing these symptoms contact the Herpes Resource Center, a nonprofit group with more than 30,000 members, based in Palo Alto, California. Some people feel that reducing consumption of caffeine, alcohol, and recreational drugs like marijuana keeps down the number of repeated attacks. The average herpes sufferer sustains about three or four new attacks per year, and these seem to become less frequent and less severe as the years go by.

Except during the recurrent attacks, which are probably not going to be more than a few times a year or less, people with herpes need not withdraw from the rest of the world. You don't necessarily have to restrict your sexual partners to other herpes victims, but at the first sign of an outbreak, you should refrain from sexual contact with people who don't have the disease. It is only fair to inform your sexual partners that you have herpes and to give the facts about contracting them. If you are married to or live with an uninfected person, don't share towels or clothing with them during your outbreaks, and wear underwear when sleeping.

Some people suffer no more than minor itching and burning with herpes, whereas others experience an agony of pain. For women in particular, urination can often burn intensely, and mere contact with fabrics can be unbearable. Many suggestions for remedies exist, such as blowing air from a hair dryer on the blisters, bathing them with a dilute iodine solution, using a topical anesthetic such as lidocaine (Xylocaine), and rinsing them with baking soda, Burow's solution, or Epsom salt dissolved in cold water. Virtually all experts agree that you should avoid clothing like panty hose (or cut out the crotch) and tight jeans and give the infection as much breathing room as possible. Drinking extra fluid helps too because it dilutes the acidity of urine and makes it less painful to urinate past any open sores.

A major concern with herpes is during pregnancy, when the virus may be transmitted to the unborn baby. At the time of delivery, after the membranes have ruptured, approximately half of the infants whose mothers have active herpes will become infected. About 1000 babies per year are born with herpes. Half of these infected infants will die, and the other half are likely to become severely affected with brain damage. Any pregnant woman, especially near term, with a history of herpes should watch herself carefully for recurrent symptoms. The doctor should perform periodic cultures of the cervical mucus, since impending infections sometimes show up in cultures before they actually show up on the body. The pregnant woman's husband or partner should be watched carefully at the same time. If a herpes infection occurs at or near delivery, the baby should be delivered by cesarean section before the membranes rupture.

Many drugs have been used to treat patients with herpes with little success. Cortisone, which is found in several over-the-counter creams, is one of these, and we believe it should be avoided, since the infection could be worsened and not relieved.

Table 13-1 Topical therapy for genital herpes

Agent	Comments
Burow's solution	Soothing for local relief only
Povidone iodine douche (Betadine)	2 teapoons of Betadine per quart of warm water
Povidone iodine sitz bath (Betadine)	4 oz of Betadine solution in a warm tub two or three times per day
Acyclovir 5% (Zovirax)	Apply every 3 hours for 7 days

Medications used to treat genital herpes are shown in Table 13-1. In 1982 a new type of antiviral ointment called acyclovir (Zovirax) was marketed to treat people infected with genital herpes for the first time. It should be emphasized that only with the first outbreak can acyclovir work. While protecting her hands with plastic gloves, the herpes victim should apply the ointment to her skin lesions every 3 hours for a week. The ointment contains a chemical that is thought to interfere with the way the herpes virus multiplies. So far the major result achieved with acyclovir is shortening of the healing process and pain episodes. Both oral and intravenous forms of acyclovir are being tested by the FDA. The hope is that these forms of the drug will be more potent and, if administered at the correct time, will kill the virus before it establishes itself in the spinal nerve roots.

Attempts are now being made to develop a herpes vaccine using a virus protein to trigger the natural defenses of the body. This vaccine would work in a preventive capacity, like smallpox or polio vaccines, and be given to the people at risk to protect them during future encounters with herpes. Preliminary work done on the vaccine appears promising, although a good deal of testing is needed before it can be made widely available.

Venereal warts

Wartlike growths called condyloma acuminatum sometimes grow on the vulva and the perineum, the area between the vaginal opening and anus. These warts are fairly common and are caused by the papovavirus. They are highly infectious and easily transmitted to sexual partners.

The usual treatment for venereal warts is the application of a liquid styptic agent called podophyllin. The compound is painted

Table 13-2 Recommended medications for uncommon genital sores

Disease	Drug
Granuloma inguinale (agent: *Calymmatobacterium granulomatis)*	Tetracycline or erythromycin
Chancroid (agent: *Haemophilus ducreyi)*	Sulfonamides (sulfisoxazole)
Lymphogranuloma venereum (agent: *Chlamydia trachomatis,* subgroup A)	Sulfonamides (sulfisoxazole, sulfadiazine), tetracycline, or doxycycline hyclate

on the small warty growths and then washed off. A few growths at a time are treated on a semiweekly or weekly basis until they are gone. Podophyllin should be used with caution under the supervision of a physician because, if it is absorbed through the vaginal mucous membrane, it can cause severe toxic effects. It should not be used during pregnancy, especially early on, because absorption could harm the fetus also.

If these warts are very extensive or if use of podophyllin is out of the question, they can be burned off or removed surgically.

Syphilis

Syphilis is one of the more dangerous and ancient of venereal diseases. It is caused by *Treponema pallidum,* a spiral-shaped bacterium. Men may notice a sore in the genital area when they have syphilis, but women may notice absolutely nothing, since their sores may be internal. The ulcers of syphilis are painless and can develop on the vulva, vagina, or cervix. Without treatment these ulcers subside, and a raised red rash on the body, especially the palms, appears. The disease is highly contagious during either of these stages. From there the disease enters a latency period in which there are no symptoms, and the only way to detect it is through the VDRL or RPR blood tests.

First- or second-stage syphilis is easily treated with penicillin using a 2.4 million unit dose of benzathine penicillin. Beyond the second stage the disease becomes more refractory, and more penicillin shots are necessary. If left untreated, it can cause blindness and severe brain damage in both the mother and the fetus. Alternate drugs that can be used instead of penicillin include and erythromycin during pregnancy and tetracycline or erythromycin when not pregnant.

Other sources

Other infectious organisms can cause genital sores, and they are listed in Table 13-2. These organisms are rare in the United States and are most commonly found in tropical climates. A skin biopsy is often necessary for definitive diagnosis of the specific disease organism. They are generally treatable with sulfa antibiotics or tetracycline.

Vaginitis

Vaginitis is the most common genital infection in women. The most common forms of infectious vaginitis include moniliasis, or yeast infections, trichomoniasis, which is a parasitic infection, and those caused by *Gardnerella vaginalis,* which are bacterial. The most common of these is moniliasis, the yeast infection.

Virtually all forms of vaginitis are characterized by an itching or burning discharge. *Trichomonas* creates a frothy, greenish discharge with a foul odor; yeast infections produce a characteristic "cottage cheese" lumpy appearance. If you notice any type of abnormal vaginal discharge, it is wise to consult your gynecologist for treatment. He or she will give you a pelvic examination and check the pH of your vaginal canal. There are, of course, normal bacteria in the vagina at all times, and they appear on the acid end of the pH scale (3.5 to 4.2). When the pH of the vagina goes above 4.2, *Trichomonas, Monilia,* and *Gardnerella* organisms have a better chance of thriving and are likely to be present.

The doctor will then examine your vaginal secretions under a microscope to inspect the organism. Yeast form little branches and buds and have a treelike appearance under microscopic examination. *Trichomonas* parasites have small tails called flagellae that whip about. *Gardnerella* organisms form clusters of debris called clue-bodies on the vaginal cells.

Many women who have these infections show few or no symptoms. Apparently there are no real hazards associated with chronic vaginal infections, but they can flare up periodically and become a nuisance. Therefore we recommend that they be treated even if they do not produce symptoms, if for no other reason than to prevent their spread to other people.

Candidiasis (moniliasis; yeast infection)

Yeast infections may cause few or no sensations when present because there are few nerve endings in the vagina to transmit them. It is only when the discharge reaches the vaginal opening and the sensitive labia that itching, redness, and soreness develop. The discharge itself has a white, lumpy appearance, often said to resemble cottage cheese. Certain conditions that change the normal pH of the vagina are linked to yeast infections. Pregnancy, oral contraceptives, diabetes mellitus, oral-genital sex, antibiotics, and excessive sweating have all been associated with yeast infections. We often advise women to insert some form of antiyeast medication into the vagina if they take antibiotics for more than 10 days.

The most effective and safest drugs available against yeast infections are clotrimazole and miconazole (Table 13-3). They rarely have adverse effects but occasionally precipitate local irritation, burning, and redness. These drugs, which come in suppository form, are usually taken in 1-week courses but may be necessary for as long as 3 or 4 weeks. Sexual partners need not be treated with the drug unless they are also obviously infected. Condoms are advisable during intercourse while the infection is still active. Home remedies such as baking soda douches and placing yogurt in the vaginal canal sometimes help treat yeast infections if they have not taken too strong a hold.

Trichomoniasis

Trichomonas vaginalis causes not only vaginal itching but also a greenish or grayish frothy discharge with a foul smell. The infection may also be the cause of certain urinary tract problems.

Table 13-3 Drugs used in the treatment of vulvovaginal candidiasis

Drug	Dosage
Miconazole nitrate 2% (Monistat 7 Cream, Monistat 7 Vaginal Suppositories, Micatin Cream)	1 applicatorful or suppository intravaginally at bedtime for 7 days; or apply cream two times per day for 2 weeks
Clotrimazole (Gyne-Lotrimin 1% Cream and Tablets, Lotrimin)	1 applicatorful or 1 tablet intravaginally at bedtime for 7 to 14 days
Nystatin (Korostatin, Mycostatin, Hilstat)	1 or 2 vaginal tablets every night for 2 weeks

Even if the infection has not been causing any symptoms and is discovered during a routine examination, both the woman and her partner should be treated. The drug used to treat trichomoniasis is metronidazole (Flagyl); for it to be effective, both partners must take the recommended dosage of 1 tablet three times per day for 7 days. A single dose of four tablets, totalling 2 gm, may be taken instead if there is some difficulty following the other regimen. Generally, we do not recommend douching, but a cleansing solution containing diluted povidone-iodine (Betadine) may be used sparingly.

Most people suffer no side effects from metronidazole, but when it is taken in large quantities, nausea, vomiting, abdominal cramping, and diarrhea may result. Never drink alcoholic beverages at the same time you take metronidazole. If you have a blood disorder or central nervous system disorder or it is early in your pregnancy, you should not use this drug. It can cause a decrease in the number of white blood cells and lead to confusion, dizziness, weakness, and irritability. It is suspected of being harmful to a fetus during the first few months of development, but this has never been proved.

Gardnerella vaginalis infection (nonspecific vaginitis)

Like *Trichomonas, Gardnerella* is a sexually transmitted organism. The first noticeable symptom is a foul-smelling discharge that causes itching or burning. This discharge and odor are usually less offensive than those caused by *Trichomonas* and

Table 13-4 Treatment for *Gardnerella vaginalis* infection

Drug	Dosage
Systemic	
Ampicillin	500 mg orally every 6 hours for 5 to 7 days
Cephalexin (Keflex)	500 mg every 6 hours for 6 days
Tetracycline	500 mg orally every 6 hours for 7 days
Metronidazole (Flagyl)	500 mg orally every 6 hours for 7 days
Local	
Sulfonamide cream (Sultrin)	Apply intravaginally two times per day for 10 days
Sulfanilamide, allantoin, and aminacrine cream (Vagitrol, AVC)	1 applicatorful or suppository once or twice per day for one menstrual cycle

are more whitish or yellowish. The most effective treatment is a 1-week course of either ampicillin or metronidazole (Table 13-4). Other effective drugs are cephalexin (Keflex), tetracycline, and sulfa creams. Both the woman and her sexual partner will need to be treated for the full week if she has nonspecific vaginitis.

Some physicians have argued that only metronidazole is 99% effective against nonspecific vaginitis, with other antibiotics running a distant second in their rate of cure. However, metronidazole is a powerful drug with potential side effects, and nonspecific vaginitis has few or no serious health consequences. Therefore the hazards versus the benefits need to be weighed before it is used to treat this infection.

Gonorrhea

Although it has not received as much recent publicity as herpes, gonorrhea also exists in the U.S. population in epidemic proportions. Controlling it is difficult because it is often undetectable in women, and men may notice only a painful discharge when they urinate. Most gonorrhea infections found in women confine themselves to the cervix, the vagina, or the bladder. Sometimes it will cause a vaginal discharge or burning during urination. If not treated, the gonorrhea bacteria may ascend up through the cervix and uterus and invade the fallopian tubes, causing a dangerous condition known as pelvic inflammatory disease. Under these circumstances the tubes can fill with pus, become plugged, and ultimately scar. Gonorrhea infections are one of the major causes of sterility in women.

There is reason for added concern when gonorrhea occurs during pregnancy. If the organism contacts the baby's eyes during delivery, the bacteria can cause a severe infection called conjunctivitis. For this reason state laws require that silver nitrate drops or erythromycin ointment be routinely put in the eyes of newborn babies.

Table 13-5 lists drugs used successfully in treating uncomplicated gonorrhea in the doctor's office. Penicillin remains the standard treatment for successfully eradicating the organisms. Initially the doctor injects penicillin in each buttock, and concurrently prescribes oral probenecid, a drug that prolongs the effectiveness of penicillin. Unfortunately, certain people are allergic

Table 13-5 Treatment of vaginal gonorrhea infections

Treatment of choice
  Aqueous procaine penicillin G, 4.8 million units intramuscularly, with 1 gm probenecid orally
  Tetracycline hydrochloride, 500 mg orally four times per day for 5 days
Slightly less effective
  Ampicillin, 3.5 gm, with 1 gm probenecid orally
  Amoxicillin, 3.5 gm, with 1 gm probenecid orally
For penicillin treatment failures or penicillin allergies
  Spectinomycin, 2 gm intramuscularly (one dose)

to penicillin and develop hives, difficulty in breathing, or a fast heart rate when they take it. Spectinomycin can be used as an alternate antibiotic.

Sexual partners should receive the same course of treatment. A week or so after therapy the physician will obtain a culture specimen from the secretions from the cervix and rectum to determine if the drug course was effective.

Pelvic inflammatory disease

Pelvic inflammatory disease is indeed a serious condition. If infection reaches the fallopian tubes, sterility can result from tubal blockage and scarring. The woman may experience appreciable pelvic pain as well. Inflammation of the tubes and ovaries can be caused by a variety of organisms, both sexually and nonsexually acquired, but gonorrhea is the most common cause. Other bacteria that cause pelvic infections are *Escherichia coli* (the organism most commonly found in the bowel), *Chlamydia trachomatis,* and streptococcal bacteria. Tuberculosis is known to cause pelvic inflammatory disease, but it is not seen as frequently in the United States as it was 40 or 50 years ago.

Women are most vulnerable to pelvic inflammatory disease after their periods, after having a baby, or after a D&C. The cervical mucus barrier is gone at these times, and the bacteria may ascend more easily into the uterus and fallopian tubes. Menstrual blood and tissue are ideal media for the growth of bacteria.

Extensive infection of the uterus, ovaries, and especially the fallopian tubes causes marked pelvic tenderness, fever, and an abnormal vaginal discharge. A complete blood count and appro-

Table 13-6 Antibiotics and treatment schedules for acute pelvic inflammatory disease

Treatment	Medication	
	First choice	**Alternate**
Outpatient	Procaine penicillin G, 4.8 million units, or ampicillin, 3.5 gm, or amoxicillin, 3 gm orally; each with 1 gm probenecid followed by ampicillin or amoxicillin, 500 mg four times per day for 10 days, or tetracycline, 500 mg orally four times per day for 10 days	
Inpatient (hospital)	Aqueous penicillin G, 20 million units per day intravenously, until improvement; then ampicillin, 500 mg orally four times per day to complete 10 days of therapy	Tetracycline, 250 mg intravenously every 6 hours until improvement; then 500 mg orally four times per day to complete 10 days of therapy

priate cultures must be taken. It may be necessary to insert a long needle through the upper vagina to withdraw any pus within the lower pelvis for culture. As with many other genital infections, sexual partners should also be evaluated and treated to prevent reinfection.

Because the bacteria causing pelvic inflammatory disease are inside the fallopian tubes, it is much more difficult for the doctor to obtain culture specimens and identify the specific organism to be treated. A broad-spectrum antibiotic or several antibiotics may be necessary to rid a woman of her infection. The primary antibiotic for treating pelvic inflammatory disease is penicillin, either with or without another broad-spectrum antibiotic. The favored antibiotics for treatment of pelvic inflammatory disease are shown in Table 13-6. A woman will need to be hospitalized if she does not improve after 2 days of drug treatment or if she has a pelvic mass, a temperature exceeding 100° F, or marked pelvic tenderness.

Intrauterine devices appear to have a slight correlation with pelvic inflammatory disease. The device itself somehow renders conditions in the uterus more susceptible to infection by causing an inflammation (not infection) in the uterine lining. Women with IUDs who contract pelvic infections should receive antibiotic therapy and then have their IUDs removed.

Most of the time antibiotics are effective against pelvic inflammatory disease. They relieve symptoms and eradicate the organisms at the source of the infection. Some women continue to have persistent or recurrent pelvic infections, a process that occasionally goes on for months or even years. The antibiotics simply might not attain high enough concentrations in the tissues to destroy all the bacteria present, or the bacteria become resistant to the antibiotic. As a result, women feel persistent pelvic pain, especially during sexual activity. Laparoscopy may be necessary to better assess the nature of the chronic pain and to determine whether there are other abnormalities involving the ovaries or tubes.

■ Personal experience

Debra T, a lively 28-year-old executive secretary, visited her doctor because she feared she had contracted herpes from her boyfriend. They had met at a health spa 3 months previously, and their relationship had developed to the point where they lived together on weekends. Debra had noticed some vaginal itching and blisterlike bumps in her genital area. Her gynecologist examined her and told Debra she believed that she was suffering from genital warts rather than herpes. Debra felt somewhat better because she learned that the warts were more treatable and did not recur unpredictably, as herpes did. The doctor also suspected that the cottage cheese-like vaginal discharge Debra had was the result of a yeast infection caused by *Candida albicans.*

To Debra's dismay, she learned that her boyfriend would have to be treated also. Although embarrassed and at first reluctant to tell him, Debra came to realize that her own problems would not be cured if he remained infected.

The doctor prescribed Monistat, a suppository cream, to handle the yeast infection. After 7 days of use, Debra was certain the infection had disappeared completely. Her doctor painted Podophyllin on her warts, waited 15 minutes, and then rinsed the area thoroughly. The warts gradually disappeared over a 3-week period. Debra's boyfriend consulted a dermatologist, who confirmed that a "pimple" on his penis was indeed a small wart cluster. He, too, used Podophyllin sparingly to rid himself of the warts.

Their relationship cooled somewhat after the wart incident, but they still continued to see each other occasionally. Taking the doctors' advice, they protected themselves with foam and condoms when they had sex together.

THINGS TO REMEMBER

1. The most common sites of female reproductive tract infections are the vulva, vagina, and cervix. Many viral, bacterial, and fungal infections produce no symptoms. Patient complaints typically include genital sores, vulvar itching, and vaginal discharge, which may have a bad odor.
2. Noninfectious causes may explain the vulvar itching or vaginal discharge, so a thorough history and physical examination by your doctor is necessary if symptoms persist.
3. Herpes virus infections of the genital tract usually involve the type II virus, which is sexually transmittable. Blisters and ulcers that appear for the first time may be treated effectively with acyclovir.
4. On the whole, herpes still remains difficult to treat and, once contracted, may be with an individual permanently. It is important to refrain from sexual contact during an outbreak, and to inform your sexual partners that you have herpes. Generally, unless you have an outbreak, you will not transmit herpes to another person.
5. A herpes vaccine is being developed and tested in human subjects but probably will not be available to the general public for several years.
6. Most inflammations of the vagina result from either *Candida* (yeast), *Trichomonas,* or *Gardnerella vaginalis* infections. None of these poses a threat to a woman's health, but all can be uncomfortable and cause itching, burning, and a foul-smelling discharge. The recommended drugs taken for an appropriate length of time should successfully eradicate these infections.
7. If an infection is sexually transmitted (herpes, gonorrhea, syphilis, trichomoniasis, or *Gardnerella),* certain precautions should be taken. Have your doctor search for any other

concurrent venereal infections; have your sexual partners as well as yourself treated with appropriate drugs to prevent reinfection; and have yourself reexamined after therapy to determine whether the drugs you took were truly effective.

8. Inflammation of the uterus, ovaries, and especially the fallopian tubes can be caused by many organisms, not just gonorrhea, although this is the chief cause. Rapid and adequate drug therapy is necessary to decrease the risk of pelvic abscess formation, pelvic pain, and sterility. Penicillin or a penicillin-like drug in combination with another broad-spectrum antibiotic is usually given. Hospitalization may be necessary.

14 Drugs for Urinary Tract Problems

Although they are not reproductive organs, the bladder and other lower urinary tract structures are located directly in front of the vagina, cervix, and uterus, and the two organ systems often have an impact on each other (Fig. 14-1). Problems related to difficult urination occur frequently and usually involve infection or an inability to control urination. They are a leading cause of unscheduled visits to the doctor's office. Women are more prone to urinary tract infections because they have a much shorter urethra (tube that brings urine out from the bladder), and bacteria can easily ascend the short urethra into the bladder to multiply.

Urinary tract infections

Urinary tract infections, sometimes jokingly referred to as "honeymoonitis," are in fact a very unamusing problem for women. They are somewhat rare in women who have not begun to engage in sexual activity, and an initial urinary tract infection often accompanies the first intercourse; hence the term honeymoonitis. The thrusting motion of the penis traumatizes the urethra and pushes bacteria from the outer genitals into the urethra, where they can begin to grow and move quickly up into the bladder. One preventive measure is to empty the bladder after intercourse to flush out any bacteria that might have entered.

Increased sexual activity can precipitate the problem, but it has several other causes too. Among them are surgery, pregnancy, catheterization of the bladder, improper hygiene, abnor-

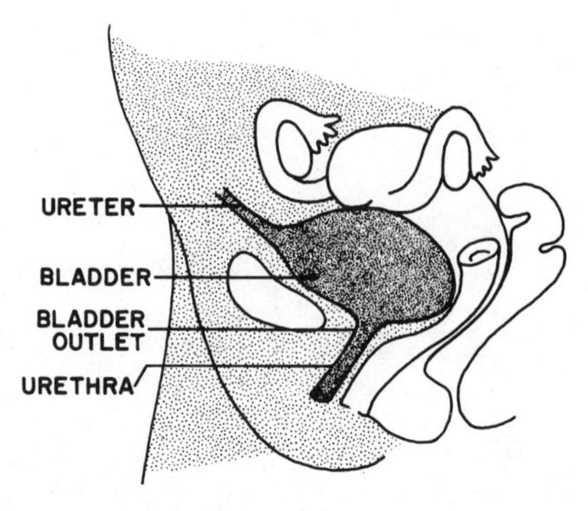

FIG. 14-1 Relation of lower urinary tract structures to the vagina, cervix, and uterus.

mal anatomy, restrictive clothing, and even failure to urinate frequently enough.

A pregnant woman is prone to urinary tract infections because her urine collecting system is somewhat static or slowed down because of the influence of hormones as well as the mechanical pressures caused by the growing fetus. From 5% to 8% of all pregnant women have a urinary tract infection with no symptoms. This problem should be treated quickly because it can turn into a kidney infection, which is more serious. Inflammation of the kidneys can precipitate premature labor, among other things. Such kidney infections tend to occur during the fifth to seventh month of pregnancy, when the uterus moves out of the pelvis and puts more pressure on the right ureter (urine collecting tube), causing poor drainage. This then makes the kidney vulnerable to bacteria if there are any in the urinary tract. Fortunately, it is usually easy to clear up urinary tract infections quickly with antibiotics.

Symptoms

The symptoms of a urinary tract infection are noticeable and often extremely uncomfortable: the feeling that you need to urinate all the time; cramping pain and burning on urination; very little actual urine production and a dark concentrated urine; and, at times, bleeding. If you have these symptoms, the best thing to do is drink large amounts of fluid, particularly water or orange or

Table 14-1 Antibiotics used to treat urinary tract infections

Drug	Dosage
Ampicillin	500 mg orally every 6 hours for 10 days
Sulfisoxazole (Gantrisin)	1 to 2 gm orally four times per day for 10 days
Tetracycline	500 mg orally every 6 hours for 10 days
Trimethoprim (Proloprim)	100 mg orally every 12 hours for 10 days
Trimethoprim sulfamethoxazole (Bactrim, Septra)	2 tablets every 12 hours for 10 days
Methenamine (Mandelamine)	1 gm four times per day for 10 days
Nitrofurantoin (Macrodantin)	50 to 100 mg orally four times per day for 10 days

cranberry juice. The high acid content of the latter two beverages has an antibacterial action. If the infection does not clear up quickly, a fast trip to the doctor's office is in order.

Treatment

Along with taking a careful medical history, the doctor will give you a thorough abdominal and pelvic examination. He or she will look for white blood cells and bacteria in the urine, a relatively simple procedure that can be done in the office. A urine specimen may be sent to a laboratory so that a culture of whatever organisms are growing in it can be done, but the doctor will probably not wait for the results to prescribe an antibiotic, probably ampicillin, one of the sulfa drugs such as sulfisoxazole (Gantrisin), or possibly trimethoprim (Table 14-1). Immediate treatment is necessary to relieve the discomfort of symptoms and to prevent the infection from spreading further into the bladder or to the kidneys. Fortunately, these drugs rapidly achieve high concentrations in urine and usually relieve symptoms within 24 hours. Drinking large amounts of fluid should accompany the antibiotic therapy; the equivalent of 6 or more glasses of water per day should be consumed.

In 95% of bladder infections the bacterium involved is *Escherichia coli,* which responds quite successfully to the drugs cited in Table 14-1. *E. coli* organisms are found in the bowel, where they are a normal rather than an infectious organism. They can find their way into the bladder when women are not careful about hygiene after bowel movements, and it is good to be conscious of this potential problem.

Recurrent infection

Most bladder infections can be successfully treated without further difficulty. They sometimes persist or recur if women fail to take the full course of antibiotics (usually four times per day for a minimum of 10 days), if an ineffective drug was prescribed to treat the specific organism, if the length of antibiotic therapy was inadequate (more stubborn infections may need to be treated for as long as a month), or if an incorrect diagnosis was made and the real problem was related to an upper urinary tract infection, menopausal changes, noninfectious inflammation, or kidney stones. Further efforts must then be made to determine the problem. The urine culture should be repeated and perhaps an x-ray examination of the kidneys, bladder, and urine collecting tubes done. This x-ray examination is called an intravenous pyelogram, or IVP. Kidney function blood tests should be performed and, if indicated, a cystoscopy. A cystoscope is a long, narrow, hollow tube with a tiny light on the end of it that allows the doctor to look at the inside of the bladder.

In women who are beyond menopause, irritation on urination may result from a loss of estrogen support for the bladder, bladder outlet and vaginal tissues. Oral estrogen pills or application of estrogen cream in the vagina may help to strengthen the bladder tissue.

Prevention

All women are well advised to take measures to prevent urinary tract infections. The primary action is to urinate at least once every 2 hours. Retaining urine causes it to concentrate, and the likelihood of infections becomes greater. A full bladder also puts pressure on the pelvic organs, causing irritation. Second, clothing that permits air circulation around the bladder and vaginal openings can prevent problems. Bacteria thrive in warm, moist, cramped environments created by tight jeans or pantyhose, particularly if they are made of synthetic fabrics rather than cotton. Panties with cotton crotches should always be purchased. Some women find that panty liners or minipads are good substitutes for undergarments that do not come with cotton crotches. Good personal hygiene, which includes daily bathing with mild soap and water and proper cleansing after urination or bowel movements, is essential. Don't, however, take bubble baths if recurrent urinary tract infections bother you; the substances in bubble baths are irritating to the delicate tissues in the female genital area. Always wipe yourself from front to back to avoid contaminating the bladder and vaginal outlets. Finally, adequate fluid consumption, that is, 6 or more glasses of water per day, is wise to promote frequent urination and keep urine from becoming too concentrated.

Urinary incontinence

Urinary incontinence is the involuntary loss of urine. This embarrassing and distressing situation occurs most frequently in elderly women in whom the nerve pathways from the brain or spinal cord to the bladder have begun to deteriorate. Another cause in the elderly is a stretching or slipping down of the opening to the bladder because of inadequate elasticity. In younger women incontinence is usually associated with the stress of laughing, running, jumping, lifting, bending, coughing, vomiting, or late pregnancy. A particular kind of neurological problem that produces uncontrollable bladder contractions is termed *urge incontinence.*

Sanitary napkins, diapers, or some other form of protection should be worn until effective medical treatment can be found for the particular form of incontinence from which a woman suffers.

Evaluation

When investigating the causes of urinary incontinence, the doctor needs a detailed history of all medical problems, particularly factors such as nervous system disorders, diabetes, and psychological disturbances. Any medications being taken should be reported, and caffeine and alcohol consumption habits should be mentioned also. The relationship of urinary tract problems to previous pregnancies or surgery must be determined.

The pelvic examination includes inspection of the top of the vaginal wall and a search for any fistula (opening or canal that would not normally be there) between the bladder and the vagina or diverticulum (outpouching) of the urethra. Muscle tone and sensation surrounding the vagina and lower bladder region must be assessed.

A woman may be asked to urinate into a special receptacle by which the doctor can determine how quickly urine is expelled and how much is retained in the bladder. A catheter is then in-

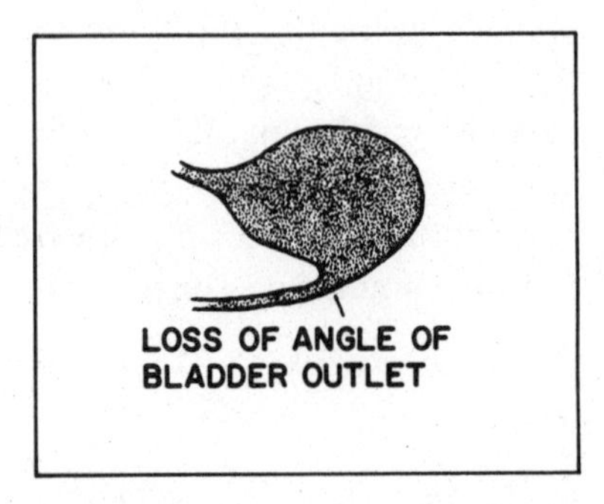

FIG. 14-2 A common cause of urinary incontinence is a distortion or loss of the angle of the bladder outlet.

serted to measure the amount of urine left. The doctor will then fill the bladder artificially using colored water. Once the bladder is full, the catheter is removed, and the vaginal canal is inspected for any staining. The presence of stain suggests a fistula. The patient is then asked to bear down so the doctor may observe any leakage. Finally, a clean cotton swab is placed in the urethra. *Stress incontinence* (Fig. 14-2) is suspected if the swab is deflected upward during the process of bearing down. Additional tests that might be made are an intravenous pyelogram, a urine culture, blood tests to check for diabetes, and possibly cystoscopy.

Treatment

Treatment depends on cause. In most cases of incontinence there is a distortion of the bladder outlet. Most affected women require a "sling" operation to lift up the outlet to restore normal anatomy. Under less extreme circumstances, or when the cause is not related to a distorted outlet, certain drugs may prove useful (Table 14-2). These medications act primarily to partially inhibit the nerves that cause contractions of the bladder and thus prevent the loss of urine. Occasionally these drugs cause dryness of the mouth, blurred vision, constipation, and weakness.

In menopausal women, once again, estrogen therapy may improve the condition of the bladder outlet by improving its blood supply and increasing its muscle tone.

Table 14-2 Drugs that aid in the storage of urine

Drug	Dosage
Propantheline (Pro-Banthine)	15 to 30 mg orally three or four times per day
Methantheline (Banthine)	50 to 100 mg orally three or four times per day
Dicyclomine (Bentyl)	10 to 20 mg orally three or four times per day
Imipramine (Tofranil)	25 to 50 mg orally three or four times per day
Oxybutynin (Ditropan)	5 mg orally two to four times per day
Flavoxate hydrochloride (Urispas)	100 to 200 mg orally three or four times per day

Table 14-3 Drugs that aid in the evacuation of urine

Drug	Dosage
Bethanechol (Duvoid, Myotonachol, Urecholine, Vesicholine)	10 to 50 mg orally three or four times per day; or 2.5 to 5 mg under the skin three or four times per day
Phenoxybenzamine (Dibenzyline)	10 mg orally one to three times per day

Difficult urination

The most hazardous condition discussed in this chapter is the inability or near inability to urinate. Although losing urine through incontinence is embarrassing, it does not pose a major threat to health. But if you do not urinate, you can become ill very rapidly. Difficulty in urinating can be caused by a bladder infection, swelling of the bladder outlet after the birth of a child or after a pelvic operation, damage to spinal or peripheral nerves, or from a tumor impeding the outflow of urine. Assessment of the problem is similar to that described for both infection and incontinence.

Drugs that are helpful in the evacuation of urine are listed in Table 14-3. Medications such as bethanechol and phenoxybenzamine, which promote bladder contractions and relax the bladder outlet, act directly by stimulating nerves in the vicinity of the bladder. Drugs such as diazepam (Valium) and dantrolene act indirectly by reducing muscle tension or anxiety. Because these drugs often have side effects, women using them must be under close observation by a physician. If drug therapy does not work, women with difficult urination will have to be catheterized or learn to catheterize themselves. In some cases surgery may be necessary to solve the problem.

■ **Personal experience**

Jeannette B, a small, frail-looking 62-year-old widow, had led an active and demanding life. She owned a highly successful real estate agency and spent what free time she had left helping her two daughters with their five children.

Ever since her teens she had had back problems stemming from a swimming accident. The pain and numbness that also involved her left leg had become almost incapacitating in recent months. Her doctor had prescribed Motrin for pain relief for her back problem and also for osteoarthritis that had developed at the base of her neck. When she visited her doctor, Jeannette told him she had not been obtaining the pain relief from the Motrin that she needed.

Her doctor ordered a myelogram, an x-ray examination of the nerves of the spine, and it revealed that some of Jeannette's degenerating vertebrae were putting pressure on some specific spinal nerve roots. A neurosurgeon offered to do corrective surgery, although he pointed out to her that the operation was somewhat risky and did not always produce the desired results. Unable to tolerate her pain any more, Jeannette decided to go ahead with the operation anyway.

Postoperatively, Jeannette found herself unable to urinate and had to be catheterized for 8 days. Because of the repeated catheterizations, she developed a urinary tract infection that required a 10-day course of Ampicillin. She was also given bethanechol tablets to help stimulate urination.

The surgery was moderately successful; her shooting pains became much less frequent. However, about 2 weeks after the operation she suddenly lost all control over her urination and bowel movements. The situation was terribly embarrassing, and Jeannette was at her wits' end. She began taking Probanthine, which helped to minimize the uncontrollable urine loss, but she found that this drug produced constipation and an uncomfortable dryness in her mouth, so she switched to Ditropan, a drug similar to Probanthine but with less of the side effects Jeannette was experiencing.

Perhaps Jeannette should not have had her operation, but with the assistance of drugs and a newly manufactured adult diaper, she has adjusted to her unfortunate surgical complications. She continues to need Ditropan, but her bowel function has returned almost to normal, so she has one less problem to contend with.

THINGS TO REMEMBER

1. Lower urinary tract problems in women of reproductive age are most commonly due to infection. In women beyond menopause the major problem is urinary incontinence.
2. Most urinary tract infections can be easily and permanently treated with an appropriate 10-day course of an antibiotic that concentrates well in urine.
3. Pregnant women are especially susceptible to urinary tract infections because of hormonal and anatomical influences. These infections should be treated quickly to prevent spread to the kidneys, which can precipitate premature labor.
4. Recurrent or persistent symptoms of urinary tract infection require a more detailed history and physical examination, urine culture, and possibly x-ray examination, blood tests, and cystoscopy.
5. If urinary incontinence, an involuntary loss of urine, persists for long periods, it is probably due to a distortion of the bladder outlet. Surgery is usually necessary to correct it, but in mild or nonsurgical cases drugs may be of value.
6. Difficulty in urinating, with retention of urine, must be treated quickly. Drugs that stimulate the nerves around the bladder or that relax the muscles may be useful, but women using them must be carefully monitored. Catheterization may be the only effective solution.
7. In women at or beyond the menopause, conditions that suggest urinary tract infection or incontinence may relate to lack of adequate support from estrogen in the tissues. Estrogen pills or the application of an estrogen cream may relieve these symptoms.

15 Menopause and Estrogen Replacement

At one time menopause was not discussed in polite company. It was brought up discreetly in private parlors by the women suffering from its symptoms and looking for a bit of sympathetic advice from those who had been through it themselves. Currently it is recognized as a major health issue, affecting up to 50 million women aged 50 or over. In 15 years that number will be much higher as the women of the post-World War II baby boom reach the end of their fertile years. What is more, probably 70% of women undergoing menopause experience one or more of the symptoms it produces, although fewer than 20% actually seek medical treatment.

Symptoms of menopause

What actually happens during menopause? In simple terms, symptoms result from fluctuating and decreasing levels of estrogen, which is produced by the ovaries and other tissues. The decline of estrogen production may be nature's way of allowing the bodies of aging women to be removed from the hazards of childbearing, which becomes risky and unwise past the age of 45. Menopause can occur naturally anywhere between the late 30s and the late 50s, but the largest number of women undergo it between ages 49 and 51. Estrogen does, however, have other functions besides stimulating the release of eggs. It plays a major role in cell growth and maintenance of cell vitality. In particular, the skin and the vaginal tract need estrogen to maintain flexibility, moisture, and good tone. It works with the calcium metabolism of the body to keep bones healthy and to prevent brittleness caused by demineralization (depletion of calcium and other minerals). It has numerous other effects on various regions of the body, such as the liver, the bladder and bladder outlet, the clotting factors of the blood, the breasts, and the pituitary gland and hypothalamus. The well-known hot flushes (or flashes) of menopause are thought to result from blood vessel instability and the metabolic control mechanisms of the latter two organs responding to decreasing levels of estrogen.

In addition to hot flushes, many women find that sexual intercourse is painful because of the dryness of the walls of the vagina; some develop urinary tract problems such as painful urination or incontinence (Chapter 14). Others begin to have problems with bone fractures and arthritic complaints. Bones actually begin to shrink, and over a course of 10 or 15 years many postmenopausal women will lose up to 3 inches of their original height.

The physical and emotional disadvantages that ensue with a lack of estrogen are obvious, and women need to know that it is possible to replace their naturally occurring estrogen and relieve these problems without significant threat to their overall health and well-being.

Estrogen replacement

Over the past 20 years a great deal has been learned about the use and action of estrogens in the body. Doctors now know that estrogen compounds given for about 3 weeks out of each month followed by a week without the drug yields the best results with the fewest number of problems. Prior to starting a course of estrogen replacement, a thorough breast and pelvic examination, including a Pap smear, is mandatory.

Preparations

To relieve annoying symptoms of menopause, a physician will prescribe one of the estrogen preparations listed in Table 15-1. Conjugated estrogen tablets are the most commonly prescribed form of estrogen replacement; they contain a mixture of nine or more synthetic estrogens with a specific chemical relationship to one another. The best known of these preparations is Premarin.

Table 15-1 Estrogen preparations and strengths

Preparation	Strengths
Oral tablets	
Conjugated estrogens (Premarin, Menotabs, Ovest, and others): 50% to 60% sodium estrone sulfate and 20% to 35% sodium equilin sulfate	0.3, 0.625, 1.25, and 2.5 mg
Esterified estrogens (Menest, Femogen, Estratabs, Evex, and others): 75% to 85% sodium estrone sulfate and 6% to 15% sodium equilin sulfate	0.3, 0.625, 1.25, and 2.5 mg
Piperazine estrone sulfate (Ogen): crystalline estrone solubilized as the sulfate and stabilized with piperazine	0.625, 1.25, 2.5, and 5 mg
Combined estrogen (Hormonin)	
Hormonin No. 1: 0.135 mg estriol, 0.7 mg estrone, and 0.3 mg estradiol	
Hormonin No. 2: 0.27 mg estriol, 1.4 mg estrone, and 0.6 mg estradiol	
Ethinyl estradiol (Estinyl, Feminone, and others)	0.02, 0.05, and 0.5 mg
17*b*-Estradiol (Estrace)	1 and 2 mg
Quinestrol (Estrovis)	100 *mg*
Diethylstilbestrol (various)	0.1, 0.25, 0.5, 1, and 5 mg
Vaginal creams	
Conjugated estrogens (Premarin)	0.625 mg per gram
Piperazine estrone sulfate (Ogen)	1.5 mg per gram
Dienestrol (D V, Estraguard, others)	0.01%
Vaginal suppositories	
Diethylstilbestrol (various)	0.1, 0.5, and 0.7 mg
Estrone (A.T.V., Prinn V/S)	0.2 mg
Estradiol (0.5 mg) and testosterone (5 mg) (Test-Estrin)	

Women should be carefully monitored when they are having estrogen replacement therapy because the doses of estrogen are relatively high, although much lower than they used to be. As with oral contraceptives, the conjugated estrogens must be processed by the liver after absorption in the gastrointestinal tract and before they enter the bloodstream, and much of the hormone will be lost during this process. Therefore the amount of hormone contained in conjugated estrogen tablets is as much as five times higher than what would normally be produced by the body.

Women whose only symptoms are vaginal dryness or bladder irritation may do better using a topical estrogen cream once or twice a week. They must remember that estrogen finds its way into the system easily and can be absorbed through the vagina to produce blood levels as high as those found in women taking tablets. Therefore topical estrogen preparations must be used prudently and only according to the physician's directions.

Treatment

As a general rule, the estrogen preparation should be taken in the lowest effective dosage. If a woman still has her uterus, she should also receive 7 to 10 days of progestin treatment each month in conjunction with the estrogen tablets. For women who have had hysterectomies, the addition of progestin is not necessary. Estrogen replacement therapy must be reevaluated every 6 months and should probably not be continued for more than 2 years at a time.

The treatment program should begin with the lowest possible dosage of estrogen. For most women short-acting oral estrogens are the preferred agents.

Baseline evaluation. Past medical history is taken to determine any reason why a woman should not have estrogens (for example, breast tumors, diabetes, gallbladder disease). A thorough physical examination is given, including breast and pelvic examinations, a Pap smear, and an examination of small pieces of tissue removed from inside the uterus by endometrial biopsy.

Medication schedule. Estrogen therapy begins at the lowest possible dosage for days 1 to 25 of each month. An oral progestin such as Provera (10 mg) or Norlutate (5 mg) should be added on days 16 through 25 if the uterus is still intact. If, after 4 weeks, hot flushes and perspiration are not relieved, the estrogen dosage should increase and progestin therapy continue. Four weeks later if symptoms are tolerable, continue the same regimen for 6 months. The progestin therapy does not have to be every month; it may be every other month. If symptoms are then tolerable, with fewer hot flushes noted while off the medication, reduce the daily estrogen dosage for another 6 months. Then, if your symptoms are tolerable but still bothersome during the drug-free period, continue your present dosage. An endometrial sample may be obtained after a period of 1 year for study. Reevaluate the effects of the regimen after 6 more months. If symptoms have become tolerable and little discomfort is noted during the drug-free period, attempt to discontinue the estrogen treatment.

Cost

The cost of estrogen replacement therapy is a modest $40 to $50 per year. Certain women should add to that the cost for supplementary calcium, such as Os-Cal, to prevent loss of minerals from the bones. Supplementary calcium will run about $30 per year. Some nutritionists believe vitamin D must be taken along with calcium to expedite its absorption. A good natural source of vitamin D is cod liver oil; pills or tablets containing this are also quite inexpensive.

Results

The most common symptom of menopause, *the hot flush,* is improved gradually rather than overnight. Over the course of 6 months many women find that the flushes decrease in number and do not seem as intense or uncomfortable when they do occur.

Because the wish to relieve *vaginal dryness* and pain during intercourse may be more urgent, doctors try to treat it quickly. A fairly high dose of conjugated estrogens may be given at the start of therapy to induce vaginal lubrication and increase the blood supply to the area. Once this occurs, they may decrease the dosage of estrogen and add progestins to the treatment program.

Estrogen creams to be applied directly to the vaginal area may be used instead and appear to be as effective as tablets. Lubricants such as K-Y Lubricating Jelly may be of small help but are not as useful as estrogens. Treating vaginal dryness with estrogens apparently does not increase sexual desire, even though it decreases the discomfort that lack of natural lubrication may cause during intercourse.

Doctors may also prescribe topical estrogen for *minor difficulty in urinating.* Because estrogen increases the blood supply to the urinary tract and has a healing effect on the lining of the urethra, the problem often improves or even clears up.

Estrogens do help in the treatment of existing *osteoporosis* (brittle bones due to loss of calcium and other minerals). Some doctors believe estrogen should be given routinely to prevent osteoporosis, but others think this is unwise. If given early, estrogen therapy may help restore lost bone tissue. Supplemental calcium and vitamin D may also be helpful. Even if started when the disease has been established for 3 or more years, it seems to help decrease the number of fractures that occur.

Some women develop an *emotional uplift* while under estrogen therapy. No one has really proved that estrogen makes any long-term impact on a woman's sense of well-being, since its beneficial effects are so subtle. At this point we do not recommend it for use during psychotherapy to create an emotional uplift. Estrogen does not seem to create or worsen depression either.

More so in previous years than now, estrogen replacement therapy was associated with certain serious problems: cancer of the lining of the uterus (endometrial carcinoma), breast cancer, blood clots, gallbladder disease, diabetes, leiomyomata (fibroid tumors of the uterus), and postmenopausal uterine bleeding. The concurrent use of progestins has greatly reduced the problems with cancer and uterine bleeding, as has the reduction of the dosage of estrogen. However, it is still essential to be examined carefully and frequently by a gynecologist when you are taking conjugated estrogens. If uterine bleeding occurs, you should see a doctor at once.

The risk of low-grade *endometrial cancer* increases with the continuous use of estrogen therapy. It occurs most often when a woman takes high doses of estrogen for a prolonged period. Therefore the monthly estrogen dosage should be as low as possible and it should be interrupted with 10 days of progestin therapy to nullify any hazard. If vaginal bleeding does occur at the end of the monthly cycle, a woman needs an endometrial biopsy.

Breast tissue is sensitive to estrogen and progesterone. It is therefore natural for a woman to be concerned about any risk of *breast cancer* during hormone replacement therapy. However, most medical studies have not proved that there is added risk with such treatment, and the evidence is not strong enough for us to discourage the use of cyclic estrogen therapy, provided that it is given in low dosages. The addition of progestins to the treatment course apparently does not affect the incidence of breast cancer one way or the other. Certainly every woman receiving hormone replacement therapy should perform a breast self-examination each month and be examined by her physician regularly.

Because the dosages of estrogens used during menopause are much lower than those used in birth control pills, the risk of forming *blood clots* is apparently no greater than for women not taking the drug. But if a woman has at any time had a blood clot in the deep veins of her legs, lungs, or brain, we advise her not to take estrogen replacement drugs.

Many medical studies have concluded that there is no increased risk of *heart disease* for menopausal women using low-dose estrogens. In contrast, women 40 to 50 years of age who take birth control pills, which have higher doses of estrogen, do have a higher risk of contracting heart or blood vessel disease.

An alternative: progesterone therapy

The other major female hormone, progesterone, acts in a competitive manner with estrogen. Its effects offset or counterbalance those of estrogen. Progestins, the synthetic version of progesterone, may be used to relieve hot flushes when conditions prohibit routine estrogen treatment. These conditions include a history of breast cancer, blood clots, or uterine fibroid tumors or if she is substantially overweight.

The progestin most commonly given is medroxyprogesterone acetate (Depo-Provera) in a 150 mg injection each month. The drawbacks to progestin therapy include the need to have a monthly injection, a greater risk of vaginal dryness, irregular vaginal bleeding, mild temporary depression, and weight gain. For these reasons doctors prescribe progestin therapy for much shorter periods than they would for estrogen.

■ Personal experience

Alice C was a trim, well-dressed woman of 57 who worked as a managing editor for a large publishing house. With an embarrassed look on her face she told her doctor, "I'm afraid middle age is starting to catch up with me. My hot flashes are getting so bad I have to have the windows wide open even when it's 20 degrees outside. To make matters worse, I have arthritis in my knees and ankles and I have to wear leg warmers so the cold air doesn't bother them. The people in my office think I'm going bananas." She paused. "What's more, my sex life with my husband has really deteriorated lately. My vagina is very dry, and most of the time I don't have much interest, I just want to get it over with. We've tried K-Y Jelly, but it's messy and really doesn't help much. My arthritis just adds to the whole problem because my legs are so sore."

When her doctor examined her, she also found that Alice had some benign fibrocystic changes in her breasts. Because Alice was having so many difficulties, her doctor decided that she would put her on low-dosage estrogen pills (Premarin, 0.3 mg) even though she had these breast changes. Alice took her Premarin for the first 3 weeks out of the month along with a progestin tablet. She went off her pills for 1 week each month.

Three months later Alice's spirits were much higher. Her hot flashes were improving steadily, and her vagina was once again lubricated. She was also taking Os-Cal calcium supplements to try to halt the progress of her degenerative arthritis. Although it had not actually improved, because Alice's other problems were being treated, the arthritis seemed to bother her less.

THINGS TO REMEMBER

1. Most women experience some response to the body's gradual decline in female hormone production during menopause. Hot flushes, vaginal dryness, skin inelasticity, osteoporosis, and urinary difficulties are examples of changes occurring from a loss of tissue stimulation by estrogen.
2. Estrogen replacement treatment to relieve these symptoms and to prevent further osteoporosis usually consists of a low-dose tablet that is taken daily for 3 weeks of each month. If a woman still has her uterus, a 7- to 10-day course of progestin medication for the remainder of the month is advisable to prevent tissue buildup or cancer developing within the inner lining of the uterus.
3. Most of the hazards associated with the estrogens in birth control pills do not apply in menopausal women because the dosage of estrogen is much lower. Low-dose preparations used for 3 weeks out of the month, with one week off the drug, are not associated with increased heart disease, blood clots, or breast, ovarian, or endometrial cancer.
4. Estrogen therapy should be stopped from 6 months to 2 years after its inception, depending on a woman's symptoms and whether she has any vaginal bleeding.
5. Local treatment using a topical estrogen cream once or twice weekly may be all that is necessary to relieve local discomfort such as vaginal dryness or burning while urinating.
6. Progestins alone are an alternative for treating hot flushes if estrogens must be avoided for certain medical reasons. Although they are considered safe, they sometimes cause unpleasant side effects such as irregular vaginal bleeding, weight gain, and mild depression.

16 Drugs for Depression, Anxiety, and Insomnia

More than 20 million people in the United States have symptoms of anxiety and depression that are serious enough to warrant treatment. Twice as many women as men are clinically depressed long enough and deeply enough to need to see a doctor. Why is this so? Women are known to be more willing to come in for treatment, so it may be that the true depth of depression in men just hasn't been documented in official medical histories.

Anxiety is something virtually everyone experiences from time to time, especially considering the stresses of modern living. The past 15 years have seen major changes in women's social roles, especially in the workplace. Some have taken added responsibilities without relinquishing those at home, undoubtedly a major cause of stress with resulting depression or anxiety. In addition, recent studies of premenstrual syndrome have shown that hormonal changes during the menstrual cycle may cause temporary symptoms of depression and anxiety. Women who are not aware of the physical basis of premenstrual syndrome symptoms may have developed more profound and lasting depression because they have believed all along that there was something wrong with them.

Depression

How do you identify a major depression and distinguish it from what is simply an unhappy but passing mood that results from conflicts in a personal or family relationship, job- or school-related pressures, or hormonal shifts? If the answer to five or more of the following questions is yes, chances are you are suffering from depression and you should seek help:

1. Have you felt a general loss of interest or pleasure in your normal activities over a period of 2 weeks or more?
2. Have you felt restless, uneasy, and uncomfortable without being able to explain why?
3. Have you noticed an appetite or weight change with no apparent physical cause?
4. Are you sleeping much more or much less than you normally do?
5. Are you more easily agitated or more sluggish in responding to others?
6. Are you considerably less energetic than usual and do you tire easily?
7. Do you feel worthless, guilty, or angry at yourself for something you think you have done?
8. Do you have trouble concentrating on things?
9. Do you often think of death or suicide?

What should you do about depression? Probably the most common reaction is to do nothing, to let it happen and simply live with it until it goes away. Between 50% and 85% of the people who experience real depression recover spontaneously after perhaps 6 to 12 months of symptoms. Unfortunately, depression has a tendency to recur; even if it doesn't, up to a year is a long time to wait for recovery. If a woman is depressed, it can be very hard on family members and others around her, besides being difficult for the woman herself. Depression can foster hostility, chaos, less productive work, and even suicide attempts.

Some people are willing to seek counseling from a psychiatrist, psychologist, social worker, clergyman, or other individual skilled in handling emotional problems. This type of support can be valuable, but it usually takes a long time to uncover the cause of the depression. This is where the use of drugs may be of assistance. Drugs used to treat depression and other forms of emotional illness are called psychoactive drugs. When used appropriately, they can quickly relieve the symptoms of depression, thus allowing a counselor to work with the person more effectively. In many cases drug treatment is all that is necessary to overcome an episode of depression.

A problem in recent years has been not the underuse of psychoactive drugs, but rather their indiscriminate use without thorough understanding of their power and their potentially beneficial and harmful effects. Women should use psychoactive drugs only under the watchful eye of a physician who understands their application and who is not willing to write an endlessly renewable prescription without frequent evaluation of the patient.

Tricyclic antidepressants

The tricyclic antidepressants are used to control major depression. In common terms tricyclics are "uppers," since they elevate your mood and restore your energy and willingness to do things. Seven brands of tricyclic antidepressants are currently available in the United States (Table 16-1). These drugs are similar, although different people may have different reactions to

Table 16-1 Antidepressant drugs

Generic name (brand name)	Oral preparations (mg)	Average daily dosage (mg)
Tricyclics		
Amitriptyline (Elavil, Endep, others)	10, 25, 50, 75, 100, 150	150 to 300
Desipramine (Norpramin, Pertofran)	25, 50	150 to 250
Doxepin (Adapin, Sinequan)	10, 25, 50, 75, 100, 150	150 to 300
Imipramine (Presamine, Tofranil)	10, 25, 50; PM: 75, 100, 150	150 to 300
Nortriptyline (Aventyl, Pamelor)	10, 25	50 to 150
Protriptyline (Vivactil)	5, 10	10 to 60
Trimipramine (Surmontil)	25, 50	150 to 250
Monoamine oxidase (MAO) inhibitors		
Hydrazines		
Isocarboxazine (Marplan)	10	10 to 50
Phenelzine (Nardil)	15	15 to 75
Nonhydrazine		
Tranylcypromine (Parnate)	10	20 to 40
Combination agents		
Amitriptyline/perphenazine (Etrafone, Triavil)	2/10, 4/10, 2/25, 4/25, 4/50	
Amitriptyline/chlordiazepoxide (Limbitrol)	12.5/5, 25/10	

each one. A knowledge of their side effects is important when choosing the correct drug. The most common side effects involve sedation and anticholinergic effects (dry mouth, blurred vision, constipation). Elderly patients may also have other anticholinergic effects such as urinary retention, psychosis (a form of mental derangement), low blood pressure, and certain other heart and blood vessel problems.

It is wise to start a course of tricyclic antidepressants with the smallest effective dosage. If results are not obtained quickly, for example, improvement in sleep habits or energy, the dosage can be increased every 24 to 48 hours. By the end of 2 weeks a woman should feel noticeably better; if she does not, she may need psychiatric help along with the antidepressant drug. Drug use can continue for 3 to 6 months if her symptoms do improve. After 6 months she should have her condition reevaluated, and if her symptoms continue to lessen in intensity, the drug dosage should be decreased gradually.

Some physicians hesitate to prescribe these drugs to pregnant women. The drugs pose no known danger to the unborn baby, but as is the case with so many other pharmaceutical agents, not enough studies have been conducted to conclusively rule out any problems. They should therefore be used cautiously during pregnancy, with the lowest possible dosages given over the shortest effective time and preferably under a psychiatrist's supervision.

Overdosing, either deliberate or accidental, is a concern with the use of these drugs. Although the tricyclic antidepressants are of tremendous benefit, they can be fatal when taken in sufficient quantities. An overdose can cause high fever, high blood pressure, seizures, and ultimately coma. If a woman overdoses on a tricyclic drug, she should be immediately attended to by paramedics or emergency room personnel. Induction of vomiting by syrup of ipecac or insertion of a stomach tube through the nose may be necessary. If she can swallow activated charcoal, it may absorb some of the drug, but this should be done under the supervision of medical personnel even if she is still conscious.

Monoamine oxidase inhibitors

If tricyclics are not effective, there are alternative drugs to combat depression. Monoamine oxidase inhibitors have been found to be particularly effective in younger people with depression characterized by anxiety accompanied by many body symptoms, hypochondriasis (obsession with imagined physical illness), irritability, agoraphobia (fear of leaving the house or being in an open space), and other types of phobias (aversions or fears). The two best known monoamine oxidase inhibitors are the hydrazine phenelzine (Nardil) and the nonhydrazine tranylcypromine (Parnate).

Major side effects, especially with tranylcypromine, include insomnia, restlessness, irritability, and agitation. Women should keep in mind that these drugs can cause problems if used in conjunction with meperidine (Demerol), alcohol, and most other central nervous system depressants. They will react with tyramine-containing substances, such as chocolate, red wine, cheese, nuts, coffee, and pickled herring, to produce severe hypertension. If the hypertension is severe, the drug should be discontinued. If the blood pressure remains elevated, it should be treated with phentolamine (Regitine).

Anxiety

Anxiety is most commonly caused by life stresses, which range from interpersonal conflicts, to financial crises to natural catastrophes. The list is endless, and it seems to increase daily as life grows more complicated. Normal anxiety usually disappears when the source of the problem is resolved. Another type of anxiety, more complex and more remote in origin, stems from fear, apprehension, and nervousness without certainty of the source of these feelings. This condition is termed *free-floating anxiety*. Persons with either form of anxiety may require treatment because the symptoms are just as uncomfortable. Persons suffering from free-floating anxiety may also need prolonged psychiatric therapy to determine its ultimate source.

Ask yourself these questions. If the answer to five or more of these is yes, you may be suffering from anxiety, and you need to find relief.

1. Do you feel keyed up, tense, and apprehensive much of the time?
2. Do you experience fear, dread, or fright without knowing why?
3. Do you have unexplainable aversions to certain things or situations?

4. Are you ever overcome with panic in public places?
5. Do you constantly feel worried and overly concerned about situations around you?
6. Do you experience breathlessness, tightness of the chest, or dizziness without any apparent cause?
7. Does your heart race, and do you have sweaty palms, shakiness, and flushing?
8. Do you get uncontrollable urges to urinate or move your bowels?
9. Do your muscles get very tense, including those in your throat? Do you sometimes feel like you're choking?
10. Do you lie awake at night with thoughts racing through your head, unable to fall asleep?

Certain drugs or medical conditions listed in Table 16-2 may cause anxiety-like symptoms. When you consult a doctor because you are suffering from anxiety, he or she should be certain to rule out such a nonemotional condition as the source.

Several types of tranquilizing drugs are used to treat anxiety. They fall into the categories of benzodiazepines, barbiturates, propanediols, β-blocking agents, certain antihistamines, and the tricyclic antidepressants. A more comprehensive list of tranquilizers or antianxiety agents, including the benzodiazepines, appears in Table 16-3.

Benzodiazepines

The benzodiazepines are the most commonly prescribed drugs for anxiety. In everyday language they are called "downers," and their brand names are familiar: Valium, Librium, Tranxene, Centrax, and Serax. These drugs are best prescribed only

Table 16-2 Conditions that may create anxiety symptoms

Drug overdose	Heartbeat irregularities
Drug withdrawal	Pheochromocytoma (adrenal gland tumor)
Caffeine overuse	Premenstrual tension
Organic brain syndromes	Lung clot
Epilepsy	Angina or heart attack
Hypoglycemia (low blood sugar)	Hyperthyroidism
Chronic lung disease	Mitral valve prolapse of heart (floppy mitral valve)
Inner ear problems	Depression
Pain	Schizophrenia

Table 16-3 Antianxiety drugs

Generic name (brand name)	Oral preparations (mg)	Average daily dosage (mg)
Benzodiazepines		
Chlordiazepoxide (Librium)	5, 10, 25	15 to 100
Clorazepate dipotassium (Tranxene)	3.75, 7.5, 15	15 to 60
Clorazepate monopotassium (Azene)	3.25, 6.5, 13	13 to 52
Diazepam (Valium)	2, 5, 10	5 to 60
Lorazepam (Ativan)	1, 2	2 to 10
Oxazepam (Serax)	10, 15, 30	30 to 120
Prazepam (Centrax)	5, 10	20 to 60
Alternatives		
Propanediols		
Meprobamate (Equanil, Miltown)	200, 400	600 to 2000
Tybamate (Solacen, Tybatran)	250, 350	750 to 2500
Antihistamines		
Diphenhydramine (Benadryl)	25, 50	75 to 300
Hydroxyzine (Atarax, Vistaril)	10, 25, 50, 100	75 to 400
Tricyclic antidepressants		
Doxepin (Adapin, Sinequan)	10, 25, 50, 75, 100, 150	50 to 150

when anxiety interferes with the ability to function normally, provided that a medical condition or use of an anxiety-producing drug such as caffeine has been ruled out. Benzodiazepine drugs are particularly valuable when a person is under sudden but short-lived stress or is about to undergo a medical or surgical procedure. Stress-provoking situations should be assessed before the prescription of these medicines. The lowest possible dosage should be taken over the shortest time needed to achieve results. Women need to understand that the use of these medicines has special applications; it should not become a daily habit, accompanying the morning coffee and cigarette. Physicians should closely monitor their patients who take benzodiazepines to see that the drugs are being used correctly.

The benzodiazepines are remarkably free from side effects when used alone. In dosages higher than normally prescribed, drowsiness and problems with coordination may develop. Elderly persons have more problems with side effects. They may also become dizzy or confused and have trouble speaking clearly and coordinating their eye muscles. These drugs must not be taken with narcotic painkillers, sleeping pills, or alcohol because they may cause dangerous drowsiness and even unconsciousness. Unpredictable side effects such as irrational rage sometimes occur.

There is a small amount of evidence that babies born to women taking benzodiazepines in the first 3 months of pregnancy have a slightly higher incidence of birth defects, notably cleft palates or lips. We therefore recommend that pregnant women not take these drugs. These medications may also accumulate in high levels in nursing infants as well, so we believe they should also be avoided when a woman being treated for anxiety is breast-feeding.

Other drugs

The propanediol drugs, such as meprobamate (Miltown, Equanil), seem to hold no advantages over the benzodiazepines in relieving anxiety and often produce more problems. They have greater potential for tolerance and dependency, and withdrawal reactions can be very severe. Nor do we recommend the β-adrenergic blocking agents such as propranolol (Inderal) for control of anxiety. We feel they are being used in inappropriate circumstances, such as when giving speeches or performing or to slow down a rapid heart rate that often accompanies normal anxiety. The appropriate use of β-blocking drugs is for certain heart conditions and hypertension, not ordinary nervousness.

Occasionally antihistamines such as diphenhydramine (Benadryl) and hydroxyzine (Atarax) may relieve anxiety. Although not as effective as the benzodiazepines, they are less habit-forming and are useful when there is a history of drug abuse. The tricyclic antidepressant doxepin (Adapin, Sinequan) may be used to relieve anxiety, but only when depression coexists.

Insomnia

Difficulties in sleeping (insomnia) usually involve an inability to fall asleep, remain asleep, or experience satisfaction after sleep. Insomnia may be the most widespread complaint of people suffering from both anxiety and depression, but it is also probably the one most clearly improved with the use of drugs.

Anxious women may plead with their doctors to give them a sleeping pill so they can at least enjoy the relief of a good night's

Table 16-4 Hypnotic drugs

Generic name (brand name)	Oral preparations (mg)	Average hypnotic dose (mg)
Benzodiazepines		
Flurazepam (Dalmane)	15, 30	15 to 30
Diazepam (Valium)	2, 5, 10	5 to 20
Barbiturate		
Secobarbital (Seconal)	50, 100	100 to 200
Halogenated hydrocarbon		
Chloral hydrate (Noctec)	250, 500	500 to 2000
Carbamates		
Meprobamate (Equanil, Miltown)	400	400 to 800
Glutarimide		
Glutethimide (Doriden)	250, 500	500
Quenazolones		
Methaqualone (Quaalude)	75	150 to 300

sleep. Physicians must, however, be careful to fully understand the cause of sleeplessness before prescribing a hypnotic (sleeping drug), especially for more than a few days. Hypnotics can be difficult to give up once a person has gotten into the habit of taking them. Hypnotics are not advisable in cases of depression or serious emotional disturbances, but antidepressant drugs are usually very helpful under those circumstances.

Hypnotics are useful for the short-term treatment of insomnia resulting from stressful adjustment situations (Table 16-4). Their principal action is depression of the central nervous system. When taken to induce sleep, the benzodiazepines (Dalmane, Valium, Serax, Ativan) are considered hypnotics and are probably the safest drugs for this purpose. They produce a better quality of sleep than do barbiturates and narcotics and have less potential for dependency and overdose. Flurazepam (Dalmane) is probably the most popular sleeping drug that has been approved for that purpose by the Food and Drug Administration.

Alternative drugs that may be used as very short-term sleep-loss remedies include secobarbital (Seconal), chloral hydrate (Noctec), meprobamate (Equanil), glutethimide (Doriden), methaqualone (Quaalude), and antihistamines in certain over-the-counter remedies. Side effects from these medications involve slowing down of breathing mechanisms, but usually only with dosages greater than would be used for sedation. Addiction is possible with long-term use.

A study has been conducted in sleep laboratories on the effects of Ovaltine. Components in this beverage act on central sleep centers and can help those afflicted with insomnia. Mixed in warm milk, this may be especially helpful.

Personal experience

Mary M, 36, was an assistant manager at a local clothing and department store. She and her husband, Bill, married just out of high school. They quarreled and disagreed throughout the course of their marriage but stayed together for the sake of their two daughters, now 14 and 17. Over the past 4 years Mary and Bill's relationship grew even more strained. Bill turned to alcohol and Mary to Valium. She started to use Valium innocently enough to relieve her occasional bouts of sleeplessness. When she found out Bill was seeing a secretary at his office, she began to rely much more heavily on the drug to relieve her sadness and pain. No one was surprised when Mary sought and was granted a divorce from Bill.

Relieved to have finally severed her ties with Bill, at the same time she found she missed him and occasionally still had mixed feelings about splitting up with him. Looking at family pictures precipitated crying spells, and despite her now steady use of Valium, she would often awaken in the middle of the night thinking of him. She had difficulty taking an interest in things around her and most of the time she felt fatigued. She found herself plagued by thoughts of her own worthlessness.

Her family doctor finally decided to treat her problem with Elavil because her low mood had persisted for 4 months. He told her she had to discontinue her use of Valium before she could start taking Elavil. Her initial dosage was 50 mg per day, but she did not find relief until the doctor increased the dosage to 100 mg per day, taken at bedtime. She improved with the Elavil and soon began to sleep more easily at night. Mary also consulted a psychologist, and he recommended group therapy to her.

Mary now belongs to a close-knit group of six people who meet once a week and under the guidance of a psychologist share their problems with each other. By attending Parents Without Partners she has met people in similar situations, has gained several new friends, and is dating a man she met there. She still uses Elavil but recently decreased her dosage without any ill effects.

THINGS TO REMEMBER

1. Anxiety and depression are widespread in the United States. Twice as many women suffer from depression as do men.
2. There are several indicators of depression, the most important of which is loss of interest and enthusiasm in normal activities.
3. Depression will often resolve spontaneously after a period of 6 to 12 months, but drug therapy may shorten this time and reduce some of the stresses it creates in the interim.
4. The tricyclic antidepressants are the most popular drugs for treating depression. They occasionally produce side effects, such as dry mouth, blurred vision, and constipation, especially in the elderly.
5. If after 2 weeks of using a tricyclic antidepressant a woman does not feel better, she may need to have the drug dosage increased and her condition reevaluated. Psychiatric therapy may be necessary.
6. An alternative to tricyclic antidepressant therapy is treatment with monoamine oxidase inhibitors. They are particularly effective in young people with unusual manifestations of anxiety, such as hypochondria and irrational fears.
7. There are several indicators of anxiety, the most important of which include tenseness, apprehension, fear, inability to sleep, and physical symptoms such as shaking, racing heartbeat, tightness of the chest, and sweaty palms.
8. Certain drugs or medical conditions may cause anxiety, and they should be considered by your doctor before any other drug is used.
9. Most people suffer from anxiety caused by life stress from time to time. A more serious condition, free-floating anxiety, sometimes requires extensive counseling along with antianxiety drugs.
10. The benzodiazepines are the tranquilizing drugs most commonly used to treat anxiety. They include Valium, Librium, Tranxene, Centrax, and Serax and generally produce no major side effects.

11. Tranquilizers should be prescribed when anxiety begins to interfere with a woman's ability to function. They should never be used beyond the time actually needed to overcome or lessen symptoms.
12. Insomnia should be treated first by decreasing the intake of stimulants such as caffeine and nicotine and by using relaxation techniques and Ovaltine in warm milk at bedtime.
13. Along with the benzodiazepines, other drugs may be prescribed to induce sleep. These medicines are intended for short term therapy when getting a good night's sleep has not been possible. Prolonged periods of insomnia require careful attention to underlying emotional or medical disturbances which are not treatable by these hypnotic drugs alone.

APPENDIX

A Comparing Costs of Drugs

Billions of dollars are spent annually to purchase over-the-counter and prescription medications. The consumer can attempt to minimize expenses, especially if the medication is to be taken over a prolonged period. It is fair to ask your doctor before leaving the office whether he or she can give you samples of the drugs that were prescribed.

The price of a medication is not necessarily equal to its quality. The cost difference between brand name and generic drugs may be virtually negligible or as much as seven times greater, so it may be worthwhile to request a generic rather than a brand name drug from your physician or pharmacist. For drugs taken regularly, ask your doctor to prescribe a large quantity (such as 100 tablets or capsules) so that you can avoid extra trips to the pharmacy and charges for filling more prescriptions. Many prescription forms contain preprinted areas in which a check mark allows the druggist to either dispense it as written or substitute a drug. Government regulations suggest that the expression "this prescription will be filled generically unless physician signs the line stating 'dispense as written' " be written on all prescription forms.

Charges for prescription drugs vary widely, so shop comparatively. Ask the pharmacist for the cost of the prescription in advance, then consider a telephone call to compare the price at another pharmacy. The following table lists wholesale prices of standard drugs described in this book. The costs reported are for 100 doses and were gathered from the *February 1983 Medi-Span Pricing Guide.* The generic equivalent may not be available for all prescription drugs. These listed prices are for relative cost comparison, and the actual cost will vary from one pharmacy to another. Prices, which include a pharmacy charge for filling the prescription, should be expected to increase by 8% to 10% each year.

Service at a pharmacy is an important consideration, along with the charges for medications. The neighborhood pharmacist may provide more personal service and cost-saving advice than one at a larger, more cut-rate drugstore or department store. When purchasing a prescription medication, ask for the expiration date (when the drug is no longer certain to be effective) to be placed on the label; if you have any leftover and unexpired medication, it can be used if your doctor writes a prescription for the same medication again.

When purchasing over-the-counter preparations, be sure to look at the ingredients—you may be spending extra money on something that you don't really need. Store brand drugs often contain the same ingredients and are usually less expensive than the nationally advertised brands. Last, purchasing a preparation in large quantities or during a sale will add to your savings.

Table A-1 Costs of prescription drugs (generic and brand name) commonly taken by women

Product	Pharmaceutical company	Medication costs (per 100) to the pharmacist (not including dispensing costs and fees) ($)
Decongestants/antihistamines		
Sudafed 60 mg tablets	Burroughs-Wellcome	6.90
Pseudoephedrine HCl 60 mg tablets	Various	1.75 to 2.95
Actifed tablets	Burroughs-Wellcome	7.99
Dimetapp tablets	A. H. Robins	14.50
Ornade capsules	SK&F	19.30
Drixoral tablets	Schering	17.88
Antibiotics		
Polycillin 500 mg capsules	Bristol	26.66
Ampicillin 500 mg capsules	Various	9.75 to 21.95
Keflex 500 mg capsules	Upjohn	89.39
Cephalexin 500 mg capsules	Various	39.95 to 61.40
Vibramycin 100 mg capsules	Pfizer	134.82

Continued.

Modified from Hafner, P.E.: Cost comparisons between commonly prescribed drugs. In Rayburn, W.F., and Zuspan, F.P., editors: Drug therapy in obstetrics and gynecology, Norwalk, Conn., 1982, Appleton-Century-Crofts.

Table A-1 Costs of prescription drugs (generic and brand name) commonly taken by women—cont'd

Product	Pharmaceutical company	Medication costs (per 100) to the pharmacist (not including dispensing costs and fees) ($)
Antibiotics—cont'd		
Doxycyline hyclate 100 mg capsules	Various	49.80 to 80.84
Achromycin-V 500 mg capsules	Lederle	9.92
Tetracycline HCl 500 mg capsules	Various	3.50 to 9.90
Erythrocin 250 mg tablets	Abbott	8.91
Erythromycin stearate 250 mg tablets	Various	5.75 to 12.47
Septra tablets	Burroughs-Wellcome	24.99
Septra DS tablets	Burroughs-Wellcome	40.92
Bactrim tablets	Roche	24.96
Macrodantin 50 mg capsules	Eaton	22.02
Nitrofurantoin 50 mg capsules	Various	7.60
Gantrisin 500 mg tablets	Roche	7.32
Sulfisoxazole 50 mg tablets	Various	2.10 to 3.59
Antidepressants		
Elavil 50 mg tablets	MSD	20.61
Amitriptyline 50 mg tablets	Various	3.00 to 12.65
Tofranil 50 mg tablets	Geigy	28.68
Imipramine HCl 50 mg tablets	Various	3.00 to 12.50
Vivactyl 10 mg tablets	MSD	20.31
Sinequan 50 mg capsules	Pfizer	22.52
Antianxiety drugs		
Valium 5 mg tablets	Roche	15.52
Librium 25 mg capsules	Roche	22.10
Chlordiazepoxide HCl 25 mg capsules	Various	1.25 to 6.75
Tranxene 7.5 mg capsules	Abbott	19.53
Ativan 2 mg tablets	Wyeth	26.23
Serax 15 mg capsules	Wyeth	16.45
Miltown 400 mg tablets	Wallace	16.48
Meprobamate 400 mg tablets	Various	0.60 to 2.95
Vistaril 25 mg capsules	Pfizer	25.76
Atarax 25 mg tablets	Roerig	25.76
Hydroxyzine HCl 25 mg tablets	Various	6.75 to 10.35
Antihypertensives		
Aldomet 250 mg tablets	MSD	14.87
Apresoline 25 mg tablets	CIBA	8.98
Hydralazine 25 mg tablets	Various	1.25 to 5.00
Inderal 40 mg tablets	Ayerst	11.75
HydroDIURIL 50 mg tablets	MSD	7.68
Hydrochlorothiazide 50 mg tablets	Various	0.50 to 5.83
Diuril 500 mg tablets	MSD	7.68
Chlorothiazide 500 mg tablets	Various	3.48 to 7.65
Lasix 40 mg tablets	Hoechst-Roussel	12.45
Dyazide capsules	SKF	13.10

Table A-1 Costs of prescription drugs (generic and brand name) commonly taken by women—cont'd

Product	Pharmaceutical company	Medication costs (per 100) to the pharmacist (not including dispensing costs and fees) ($)
Insulins		
Regular U-100	Squibb	4.61/vial
Regular U-100	Lilly	6.92
NPH U-100	Squibb	5.26
NPH U-100	Lilly	6.92
Lente U-100	Squibb	5.26
Lente U-100	Lilly	6.92
Semilente U-100	Squibb	5.26
Semilente U-100	Lilly	6.92
Anticonvulsants		
Dilantin 100 mg capsules	Parke-Davis	6.82
Sodium phenytoin 100 mg capsules	Various	0.90 to 2.29
Phenobarbital sodium 32 mg tablets	Various	0.23 to 1.50
Mysoline 250 mg tablets	Ayerst	8.80
Primidone 250 mg tablets	Various	3.80 to 4.75
Tegretol 200 mg tablets	Geigy	17.52
Tridione 300 mg capsules	Abbott	9.54
Zarontin 250 mg capsules	Parke-Davis	18.19
Depakene 250 mg capsules	Abbott	20.05
β-Adrenergic tocolytic agents		
Vasodilan 10 mg tablets	Mead-Johnson	17.54
Isoxsuprine HCl 10 mg tablets	Various	3.09 to 9.25
Brethine 2.5 mg tablets	Geigy	11.51
Bricanyl 2.5 mg tablets	Astra	10.10
Yutopar 10 mg tablets	Merrell-National	61.98
Antiemetics		
Bendectin tablets	Merrell-National	38.99
Phenergan 25 mg suppositories	Wyeth	7.01
Compazine 25 mg suppositories	SK&F	8.00
Oral contraceptives		
Ortho-Novum 1/50, 21, or 28	Ortho	8.20
Norinyl 1/50, 21 or 28	Syntex	8.90
Ovral 21 or 28	Wyeth	9.35
Ovcon-50, 21	Mead-Johnson	7.39
Norlestrin 1/20, 21 or 28	Parke-Davis	8.49
Demulen 21 or 28	Searle	10.68
Ortho-Novum 1/35, 21 or 28	Ortho	8.20
Norinyl 1/35, 21 or 28	Syntex	8.90
Lo/Ovral 1/35, 21 or 28	Wyeth	9.35
Brevicon 21 or 28	Syntex	9.20
Modicon 21	Ortho	8.20
Ovcon 35, 21	Mead-Johnson	7.39
Loestrin 1/20, 21	Parke-Davis	8.49
Loestrin 1.5/30	Parke-Davis	8.49

Continued.

Table A-1 Costs of prescription drugs (generic and brand name) commonly taken by women—cont'd

Product	Pharmaceutical company	Medication costs (per 100) to the pharmacist (not including dispensing costs and fees) ($)
Drugs for pelvic pain		
Danocrine 200 mg capsules	Winthrop	116.16
Indocin 25 mg capsules	MSD	22.46
Clinoril 150 mg tablets	MSD	40.07
Naprosyn 250 mg tablets	Syntex	38.30
Anaprox 275 mg tablets	Syntex	35.33
Motrin 400 mg tablets	Upjohn	22.38
Ponstel 250 mg capsules	Parke-Davis	26.52
Bayer 325 mg tablets	Glenbrook	2.04
Aspirin 325 mg tablets	Various	0.27 to 0.99
Tylenol 325 mg tablets	McNeil	2.88
Acetaminophen 325 mg tablets	Various	0.90 to 1.75
Urologic disorders		
Urecholine 10 mg tablets	MSD	22.91
Bethanechol HCl 10 mg tablets	Various	1.65 to 12.38
Dibenzyline 10 mg capsules	SK&F	11.65
Anticholinergics/antispasmodics		
Urispas 100 mg tablets	SK&F	15.00
Enuretrol tablets	Berlex	6.60
Ditropan 5 mg tablets	Marion	17.69
Bentyl 10 mg capsules	Merrell-National	7.76
Dicyclomine HCl 10 mg capsules	Various	1.30 to 4.70
Probanthine 15 mg tablets	Searle	20.02
Propantheline HBr 15 mg tablets	Various	1.25 to 7.25
Vulvovaginal candidiasis preparations		
Mycostatin Vaginal tablets 100,000 U	Squibb	6.35
Nilstat Vaginal tablets 100,000 U	Lederle	6.07
Nystatin vaginal tablets 100,000 U	Various	1.45 to 2.30/15
Monistat-7 Vaginal Cream	Ortho	7.30/47 gm
Gyne-Lotrim 100 mg tablets	Schering	6.81/7
Gyne-Lotrim Vaginal Cream 7-day	Schering	6.48/45 gm
Mycelex-G 100 mg tablets	Dome	6.95/7
Mycelex Vaginal Cream 7-day	Dome	6.61/45 gm
Nonspecific vaginitis preparations		
Tetracycline—see Antibiotics		
Ampicillin—see Antibiotics		
Flagyl 250 mg tablets	Searle	74.46
Metronidazole 250 mg tablets	Generix	34.45
Sultrin Vaginal Cream	Ortho	9.50/78 gm
Triple sulfa vaginal cream	Various	2.50 to 4.10/78 gm

Table A-1 Costs of prescription drugs (generic and brand name) commonly taken by women—cont'd

Product	Pharmaceutical company	Medication costs (per 100) to the pharmacist (not including dispensing costs and fees) ($)
Estrogens		
Estrace 1 mg tablets	Mead-Johnson	8.47
Diethylstilbestrol 0.5 mg tablets	Various	0.65 to 1.65
Premarin 0.625 mg tablets	Ayerst	7.60
Conjugated estrogens 0.625 mg tablets	Various	1.87 to 6.82
Estrovis 100 μg tablets	Parke-Davis	30.92
Menest 0.625 mg tablets	Beecham	7.00
Amnestrogen 0.625 mg tablets	Squibb	7.20
Evex 0.625 mg tablets	Syntex	8.12
Ogen 0.75 mg tablets	Abbott	6.89
Estinyl 0.05 mg tablets	Schering	14.33
Feminone 0.05 mg tablets	Upjohn	2.51

APPENDIX

B Interactions Between Commonly Used Drugs

Drugs	Interaction
Aminoglycosides	
Cephaloridine	Increased kidney toxicity
Cephalothin	Possible increased kidney toxicity
Digoxin	Possible decreased digoxin effect
Ethacrynic acid	Increased ear toxicity (both hearing and balance or orientation)
Polymyxins	Increased kidney toxicity
Ampicillin	
Contraceptives, oral	Decreased contraceptive effect
Anesthetics, general	
Antihypertensive drug	Lowered blood pressure
Antacids	
Digoxin	Decreased digoxin levels
Indomethacin	Decreased indomethacin levels
Isoniazid	Decreased isoniazid effect with aluminum antacids
Salicylates	Decreased salicylate levels
Tetracyclines, oral	Decreased tetracycline levels
Anticoagulants, oral	
Barbiturates	Decreased bleeding risk
Carbamazepine	Decreased bleeding risk
Cimetidine	Increased bleeding risk
Contraceptives, oral	Decreased bleeding risk
Hypoglycemics	Decreased blood sugar levels
Indomethacin	Increased bleeding risk
Metronidazole	Increased bleeding risk
Miconazole	Increased bleeding risk
Phenylbutazone or oxyphenbutazone	Increased bleeding risk
Phenytoin	Increased phenytoin toxicity with dicumarol

Drugs	Interaction
Anticoagulants, oral—cont'd	
Rifampin	Decreased bleeding risk
Salicylates	Increased bleeding time
(more than 2 gm/day)	Increased bleeding risk
Sulfinpyrazone	Increased bleeding risk
Sulfonamides	Increased bleeding risk
Thyroid hormones	Increased bleeding risk
Barbiturates (all represent interactions with phenobarbital)	
Anticoagulants, oral	Decreased bleeding risk
Antidepressants, tricyclic	Decreased antidepressant effect
Chloramphenicol	Increased barbiturate effect
Contraceptives, oral	Decreased contraceptive effect
Corticosteroids	Decreased steroid effect
Digitoxin	Decreased digitoxin effect
Doxycycline	Decreased doxycycline effect
Meperidine	Increased central nervous system depression
Phenothiazines	Decreased phenothiazine effect
Propranolol	Decreased propranolol effect
Rifampin	Decreased barbiturate effect
Valproic acid	Increased phenobarbital effect
Benzodiazepines	
Cimetidine	Increased effect of chlordiazepoxide and diazepam
Cephaloridine	
Aminoglycoside antibiotics	Increased kidney toxicity
Ethacrynic acid	Increased kidney toxicity
Furosemide	Increased kidney toxicity
Cephalothin	
Aminoglycoside antibiotics	Possible increased kidney toxicity
Chloramphenicol	
Barbiturates	Increased barbiturate effect
Phenytoin	Increased phenytoin toxicity
Cimetidine	
Anticoagulants, oral	Increased bleeding risk
Benzodiazepines	Increased effect of chlordiazepoxide
Theophylline	Increased theophylline toxicity
Contraceptives, oral	
Ampicillin	Decreased contraceptive effect
Anticoagulants, oral	Decreased bleeding risk
Barbiturates	Decreased contraceptive effect
Carbamazepine	Decreased contraceptive effect

Continued.

Drugs	Interaction
Contraceptives, oral—cont'd	
Guanethidine	Decreased guanethidine effect
Hypoglycemics, oral	Increased blood sugar levels
Phenytoin	Decreased contraceptive effect
Primidone	Decreased contraceptive effect
Tetracyclines	Decreased contraceptive effect
Diazepam	Increased diazepam effect
Corticosteroids	
Barbiturates	Decreased corticosteroid effect
Diuretics	Increased potassium loss
Ephedrine	Decreased dexamethasone effect
Estrogens	Usually increased corticosteroid effect
Phenytoin	Decreased corticosteroid effect
Rifampin	Decreased corticosteroid effect
Digoxin	
Antacids, oral	Decreased digoxin effect
Diuretics	Increased digoxin toxicity
Ergot alkaloids (ergotamine, ergotrate, cafergot, and similar agents)	
Ephedrine	High blood pressure
Methoxamine	High blood pressure, headaches
Sympathomimetics	High blood pressure, headaches
Estrogens	
Anticoagulants	Usually decreased bleeding risk
Hypoglycemics	Increased blood sugar levels
Oxytocin	Increased uterine contractility
Phenobarbital	Decreased estrogen levels
Vitamins	Decreased folate levels
Furosemide	
Cephaloridine	Increased kidney toxicity
Corticosteroids	Increased potassium loss
Digitalis drugs	Increased digitalis toxicity
Indomethacin	Decreased antihypertensive effect and water loss
Lithium	Increased lithium toxicity
Phenytoin	Reduced urination
Propranolol	More decrease in heart rate and blood pressure
Heparin	
Aspirin	Increased bleeding risk
Hydralazine	
Anesthetics, general	Lowered blood pressure
Sympathomimetic amines	Decreased antihypertensive effect

Drugs	Interaction
Hypoglycemics, oral	
Contraceptives, oral	Increased blood sugar levels
Propranolol	Prolonged lower blood sugar levels Masks rapid heart rate and tremor High blood pressure during hypoglycemia
Rifampin	Decreased effect in reducing blood sugar levels
Salicylates	Lower blood sugar levels
Indomethacin	
Antacids, oral	Decreased indomethacin effect
Anticoagulants, oral	Increased bleeding risk
Diuretics	Decreased antihypertensive and water loss effect of thiazides and furosemide
Lithium	Increased lithium toxicity
Propranolol	Decreased antihypertensive effect
Sympathomimetic amines	Severe high blood pressure
Influenza vaccine	
Theophylline	Increased theophylline effect
Insulin	
Corticosteroids	Increased blood sugar levels
Diuretics (Thiazide)	Increased blood sugar levels
Oral contraceptives	Increased blood sugar levels
Propranolol	Increased insulin activity, lower blood sugar levels
Iron, oral	
Tetracyclines	Decreased tetracycline effect
Isoniazid	
Aluminum antacids	Decreased isoniazid effect
Phenytoin	Increased phenytoin toxicity
Lithium	
Diuretics	Increased lithium toxicity
Indomethacin	Increased lithium toxicity
Methyldopa	Increased lithium toxicity
Phenothiazines	Decreased phenothiazine levels
Methyldopa	
Anesthetics, general	Lower blood pressure
Lithium	Increased lithium toxicity
Tolbutamide	Lower blood sugar levels
Metronidazole	
Alcohol	Increased alcohol toxicity
Anticoagulants, oral	Increased bleeding risk

Continued.

Drugs	Interaction
Miconazole	
Amphotericin B	Decreased anticandidal effect
Anticoagulants, oral	Increased bleeding risk
Phenothiazines	
Barbiturates	Decreased phenothiazine effect
Propranolol	Increased effects of chlorpromazine and propranolol
Phenytoin	
Antidepressants, tricyclic	Increased phenytoin toxicity with imipramine
Contraceptives, oral	Decreased contraceptive effect
Corticosteroids	Decreased corticosteroid effect
Doxycycline	Decreased doxycycline effect
Furosemide	Decreased urination
Isoniazid	Increased phenytoin toxicity
Phenylbutazone	Increased phenytoin toxicity
Primidone	
Contraceptives, oral	Decreased contraceptive effect
Propranolol	
Anesthetics, general	Lower blood pressure
Barbiturates	Smaller decrease in both heart rate and lowering of blood pressure
Chlorpromazine	Increased effects of both drugs
Hypoglycemics, oral	Prolonged low blood sugar levels Masks rapid heart rate and tremor High blood pressure during hypoglycemia
Indomethacin	Decreased antihypertensive effect
Lidocaine	Increased lidocaine effect
Theophylline	Increased theophylline effect with propranolol
Ritodrine	
Anesthetics, general	Lower blood pressure
Corticosteroids	Fluid in lungs
Digitalis	Heart rate irregularities
Hypoglycemics	Increased blood sugar levels
Propranolol	Antagonism
Salicylates	
Antacids	Decreased salicylate levels
Anticoagulants, oral	Possible increased bleeding risk with aspirin Increased bleeding risk (more than 2 gm/day of salicylates)
Heparin	Increased bleeding risk
Hypoglycemics	Lower blood sugar levels

Drugs	Interaction
Sulfamethoxazole-trimethoprim	Same as sulfonamides
Sulfonamides	
Anticoagulants, oral	Increased bleeding risk
Hypoglycemics	Lower blood sugar levels
Sympathomimetic amines	
Antihypertensive drugs	Decreased antihypertensive effect
Propranolol	High blood pressure with epinephrine, possibly with others
Digitalis drugs	Increased tendency to heart rate irregularities
Tetracyclines	
Antacids, oral	Decreased tetracycline effect
Barbiturates	Decreased doxycycline effect
Carbamazepine	Decreased doxycycline effect
Contraceptives, oral	Decreased contraceptive effect
Iron, oral	Decreased tetracycline effect
Phenytoin	Decreased doxycycline effect
Theophylline	
Cimetidine	Increased theophylline toxicity
Erythromycin	Increased theophylline effect
Influenza vaccine	Increased theophylline effect
Smoking (tobacco and marijuana)	Decreased theophylline effect
Thiazide diuretics	
Corticosteroids	Increased potassium loss
Digitalis drugs	Increased digitalis toxicity
Indomethacin	Decreased antihypertensive and water loss effects
Thyroid hormones	
Anticoagulants	Increased bleeding risk
Vitamin K	
Antibiotics	Decreased clotting factor synthesis
Mineral oil	Decreased clotting factor synthesis

APPENDIX

C Generic and Brand Name Drug Cross-Reference Guide

Drugs or drug type	Brand names	Generic name
Acetaminophen (systemic)	Datril	Acetaminophen
	Liquiprin	
	Phenaphen	
	SK-APAP	
	Tempra	
	Tylenol	
	Tylenol Extra Strength	
	Valadol	
Acetaminophen and codeine (systemic)	Aceta with Codeine	
	Capital with Codeine	
	Empracet with Codeine	
	Papa-Deine	
	Pavadon	
	Phenaphen with Codeine	
	Proval	
	SK-APAP with Codeine	
	Tylenol with Codeine	
Adrenocorticoids (topical)	Cyclocort	Amcinonide
	Benisone	Betamethasone
	Celestone	
	Valisone	
	Tridesilon	Desonide
	Topicort	Desoximetasone
	Aeroseb-Dex	Dexamethasone
	Decaderm	
	Decadron	
	Decaspray	

Drugs or drug type	Brand names	Generic name
Adrenocorticoids (topical)—cont'd	Hexadrol	
	Florone	Diflorasone
	Locorten	Flumethasone
	Fluonid Flurosyn Synalar	Fluocinolone
	Lidex Topsyn	Fluocinonide
	Oxylone	Fluorometholone
	Cordran	Flurandrenolide
	Halciderm Halog	Halcinonide
	Cortaid Cort-Dome Cortef Cortisol Cortril Dermacort Hydrocortone Hytone Texacort	Hydrocortisone
	Medrol	Methylprednisolone
	Meti-Derm	Prednisolone
	Aristocort Aristogel Kenalog Spencort Triacet	Triamcinolone
Adrenocorticoids (systemic)	Celestone	Betamethasone
	Cortone	Cortisone
	Decadron Dexasone Hexadrol	Dexamethasone
	Alphadrol	Fluprednisolone

Continued.

Drugs or drug type	Brand names	Generic name
Adrenocorticoids (systemic)—cont'd	A-Hydrocort Cortef Cortenema Hydrocortone Solu-Cortef	Hydrocortisone
	Betapar	Meprednisone
	A-MethaPred Duralone Medralone Medrol Methylone	Methylprednisolone
	Haldrone	Paramethasone
	Delta-Cortef Hydeltrasol Meticortelone Sterone	Prednisolone
	Predoxine	Prednisolone, buffered
	Deltasone Meticorten Orasone Sterapred	Prednisone
	Aristocort Aristospan Cinonide Kenacort Kenalog Tramacort	Triamcinolone
	Doca Percorten	Desoxycorticosterone
	Florinef	Fludrocortisone
Alcohol and acetone (topical)	Seba-Nil Sebasum Tyrosum	
Alcohol and sulfur (topical)	Acne Aid Acnomead Epi-Clear Liquimat Postacne Transact Xerac	

Drugs or drug type	Brand names	Generic name
Allopurinol (systemic)	Lopurin Zyloprim	Allopurinol
Aminoglycosides (systemic)	Amikin	Amikacin
	Apogen Bristagen Garamycin U-Gencin	Gentamicin
	Kantrex Klebcil	Kanamycin
	Mycifradin	Neomycin, Streptomycin
	Nebcin	Tobramycin
Amphetamines (systemic)	Benzedrine	Amphetamine
	Dexampex Dexedrine Diphylets Ferndex Obotan Oxydess Spancap	Dextroamphetamine
	Desoxyn Methampex	Methamphetamine
Anticoagulants (systemic)	Miradon	Anisindione
	Hedulin	Phenindione
	Liquamar	Phenprocoumon
	Athrombin-K	Warfarin potassium
	Coumadin Panwarfin	Warfarin sodium
Antidiabetics, oral (systemic)	Dymelor	Acetohexamide
	Diabinese	Chlorpropamide
	Tolinase	Tolazamide
	Orinase	Tolbutamide

Continued.

Drugs or drug type	Brand names	Generic name
Antihistamines (systemic)	Optimine	Azatadine
	Ambodryl	Bromodiphenhydramine
	Bromphen Dimetane Puretane Symptom 3	Brompheniramine
	Clistin	Carbinoxamine
	Chloramate Chlor-Trimeton Histaspan Phenetron Teldrin	Chlorpheniramine
	Tavist	Clemastine
	Cyprodine Periactin	Cyproheptadine
	Polaramine	Dexchlorpheniramine
	Dramamine Eldodram	Dimenhydrinate
	Dimethpyrindene Forhistal Triten	Dimethindene
	Benadryl Bendylate Eldadryl Valdrene	Diphenhydramine
	Diafen Hispril	Diphenylpyraline
	Decapryn	Doxylamine
	Allertoc Mepyramine Thylogen	Pyrilamine
	PBZ Pyribenzamine	Tripelennamine
	Actidil	Triprolidine

Drugs or drug type	Brand names	Generic name
Antithyroid agents (systemic)	Tapazole Thiamazole	Methimazole
	Propacil Propyl-Thyracil	Propylthiouracil
APC (Aspirin, phenacetin, and caffeine) (systemic)	Acetophen Aidant APAC A.S.A. Compound Asalco No. 1 Asphac-G P-A-C Compound Phencaset Sal-Fayne Salphenine Tabloid APC	
APC and codeine (systemic)	Empirin Compound with Codeine A.S.A. and Codeine Compound P-A-C Compound with Codeine Salatin with Codeine Tabloid APC with Codeine	
Appetite suppressants (systemic)	Didrex	Benzphetamine
	Pre-Sate	Chlorphentermine
	Voranil	Clortermine
	Tenuate Tepanil	
	Sanorex	Mazindol
	Bontril PDM Phendiet Plegine	Phendimetrazine
	Preludin	Phenmetrazine
	Fastin Ionamin	Phentermine
Barbiturates (systemic)	Amytal	Amobarbital

Continued.

Drugs or drug type	Brand names	Generic name
Barbiturates (systemic)—cont'd	Buticaps Butisol	Butabarbital
	Sombulex	Hexobarbital
	Mebaral	Mephobarbital
	Gemonil	Metharbital
	Nembutal	Pentobarbital
	Sedadrops SK-Phenobarbital Solfoton	Phenobarbital
	Seconal	Secobarbital
	Tuinal	Secobarbital and amobarbital
	Lotusate	Talbutal
Belladonna alkaloids and barbiturates (systemic)	Minabel Omnibel Palbar	Atropine, hyoscyamine, scopolamine, and butabarbital
	Cyclo-Bell	Atropine, hyoscyamine, scopolamine, butabarbital, pentobarbital, and phenobarbital
	Barbidonna Donna-Sed Donnatal Donphen Hasp Hybephen Hyosophen Kinesed Sedralex Setamine Spalix Spasmolin Spasmophen Spasmorel Tri-Spas	Atropine, hyoscyamine, scopolamine, and Phenobarbital
	Alised Antrocol Atrobarb	Atropine and phenobarbital

Drugs or drug type	Brand names	Generic name
Belladonna alkaloids and barbiturates (systemic)—cont'd	Amobell	Belladonna and amobarbital
	Butibel	Belladonna and butabarbital
	Belap Bellophen Bello-Phen Chardonna Donabarb Donnabarb Oxoids Phenobel Phenobella Sedajen Valaspas	Belladonna and phenobarbital
	Hybar	Hyoscyamine, scopolamine, and phenobarbital
	Cystospaz-SR	Hyoscyamine and butabarbital
	Anaspaz PB Levsin-PB Levsin w/Phenobarbital Levsinex w/ Phenobarbital	Hyoscyamine and phenobarbital
Benzodiazepines (systemic)	A-poxide Librium SK-Lygen	Chlordiazepoxide
	Tranxene	Clorazepate
	Valium	Diazepam
	Dalmane	Flurazepam
	Ativan	Lorazepam
	Serax	Oxazepam
	Verstran	Prazepam
Benzoyl peroxide (topical)	Benoxyl Benzac Benzagel	Benzoyl peroxide

Continued.

Drugs or drug type	Brand names	Generic name
Benzoyl peroxide (topical)—cont'd	Clear By Design Dermodex Desquam-X Epi-Clear Fostex BPO Panoxyl Persadox Persa-Gel Porox 7 Teen Topex Xerac BP	
Beta-adrenergic blocking agents (systemic)	Lopressor	Metoprolol
	Corgard	Nadolol
	Inderal	Propranolol
Bethanechol (systemic)	Duvoid Myotonachol Urecholine	
Bleomycin (systemic)	Blenoxane	Bleomycin
Bromocriptine (systemic)	Parlodel	Bromocriptine
Brompheniramine, guaifenesin, phenylephrine, and phenylpropanolamine (systemic)	Dimetane expectorant Midatane expectorant Normatene expectorant Puretane expectorant Spentane expectorant	
Brompheniramine, guaifenesin, phenylephrine, phenylpropanolamine, and codeine (systemic)	Dimetane expectorant-DC Midatane DC expectorant Normatane DC expectorant Puretane Expectorant DC Spentane DC expectorant	
Brompheniramine, phenylephrine, and phenylpropanolamine (systemic)	Brompheniramine Compound Bromatapp Dimetapp Eldatapp Puretapp	

Drugs or drug type	Brand names	Generic name
Busulfan (systemic)	Myleran	Busulfan
Butalbital and APC (systemic)	Fiorinal	
Butalbital, APC, and codeine (systemic)	Fiorinal with Codeine	
Butorphanol (systemic)	Stadol	Butorphanol
Calcitonin (systemic)	Calcimar	Calcitonin
Carboprost (systemic)	Prostin/15 M	Carboprost
Carisoprodol (systemic)	Rela Soma Soprodol	Carisoprodol
Cephalosporins (systemic)	Ceclor	Cefaclor
	Duricef Ultracef	Cefadroxil
	Mandol	Cefamandole
	Ancef Kefzol	Cefazolin
	Mefoxin	Cefoxitin
	Keflex	Cephalexin
	Kafocin	Cephaloglycin
	Loridine	Cephaloridine
	Keflin Neutral	Cephalothin
	Cefadyl	Cephapirin
	Anspor Velosef	Cephradine
Charcoal, activated (oral)	Charcocaps Charcodote Charcotabs	

Continued.

Drugs or drug type	Brand names	Generic name
Chloral hydrate (systemic)	Aquachloral Cohidrate Noctec Oradrate	
Chlorambucil (systemic)	Leukeran	Chlorambucil
Chloramphenicol (systemic)	Amphicol Chloromycetin	Chloramphenicol
Chloramphenicol (topical)	Chloromycetin	Chloramphenicol
Chlordiazepoxide and amitriptyline (systemic)	Limbitrol	
Chlordiazepoxide and clidinium (systemic)	Librax	
Chlorpheniramine, phenylpropanolamine, and isopropamide (systemic)	Allernade Capade Ornade	
Cholestyramine (oral)	Questran	Cholestyramine
Cimetidine (systemic)	Tagamet	Cimetidine
Cisplatin (systemic)	Platinol	Cisplatin
Clindamycin (topical)	Cleocin T	Clindamycin
Clofibrate (systemic)	Atromid-S	Clofibrate
Clomiphene (systemic)	Clomid	Clomiphene
Clonidine (systemic)	Catapres	Clonidine
Clonidine and chlorthalidone (systemic)	Combipres	
Clotrimazole (topical)	Lotrimin Mycelex	Clotrimazole

Drugs or drug type	Brand names	Generic name
Clotrimazole (vaginal)	Gyne-Lotrimin	Clotrimazole
Colchicine (systemic)	Colsalide Improved	Colchicine
Colistin, neomycin, and hydrocortisone (otic)	Coly-Mycin S	
Cyclobenzaprine (systemic)	Flexeril	Cyclobenzaprine
Cyclophosphamide (systemic)	Cytoxan	Cyclophosphamide
Cycloserine (systemic)	Seromycin	Cycloserine
Cytarabine (systemic)	Cytosar-U	Cytarabine
Dacarbazine (systemic)	DTIC-Dome	Dacarbazine
Dactinomycin (systemic)	Cosmegen	Dactinomycin
Danazol (systemic)	Danocrine	Danazol
Dantrolene (systemic)	Dantrium	Dantrolene
Dapsone (systemic)	Avlosulfon	Dapsone
Dexbrompheniramine and pseudoephedrine (systemic)	Disophrol Drixoral	
Diazoxide (oral)	Proglycem	Diazoxide
Dicyclomine (systemic)	Bentyl Dyspas	Dicyclomine
Digitalis medicines (systemic)	Cedilanid-D	Deslanoside
	Digifortis Pil-Digis	Digitalis
	Crystodigin Purodigin	Digitoxin
	Lanoxin	Digoxin

Continued.

Drugs or drug type	Brand names	Generic name
Digitalis medicines (systemic)—cont'd	Gitaligin	Gitalin
	Cedilanid	Lanatoside C
	Strophanthin-G	Ouabain
Dinoprost (intraamniotic)	Prostin F_2 Alpha	Dinoprost
Dinoprostone (vaginal)	Prostin E_2	Dinoprostone
Dione-type anticonvulsants (systemic)	Paradione	Paramethadione
	Tridione	Trimethadione
Diphenoxylate and atropine (systemic)	Colonil Lomotil SK-Diphenoxylate	
Dipyridamole (systemic)	Persantine	Dipyridamole
Disopyramide (systemic)	Norpace	Disopyramide
Disulfiram (systemic)	Antabuse	Disulfiram
Doxapram (systemic)	Dopram	Doxapram
Doxylamine and pyridoxine (systemic)	Bendectin	
Drocode, promethazine, and APC (systemic)	Synalgos-DC	
Ephedrine (systemic)	Ectasule Minus Ephedsol	
Epinephrine (systemic)	Adrenalin AsthmaHaler Bronitin Bronkaid Medihaler-Epi Primatene	Epinephrine
	AsthmaNefrin microNEFRIN Vaponefrin	Racepinephrine
Ergoloid mesylates (systemic)	Hydergine	

Drugs or drug type	Brand names	Generic name
Ergonovine (systemic)	Ergotrate	Ergonovine
	Methergine	Methylergonovine
Ergotamine (systemic)	Ergomar Ergostat Gynergen Medihaler Ergotamine	Ergotamine tartrate
Ergotamine, belladonna alkaloids, and phenobarbital (systemic)	Bellergal Bellergal-S	
Ergotamine and caffeine (systemic)	Cafergot Cafermine Cafetrate Ergocaf Ergocaffeine Lanatrate Migrastat	
Ergotamine, caffeine, belladonna alkaloids, and phenobarbital (systemic)	Cafergot-PB	
Erythromycin (systemic)	E-Mycin Ilotycin Robimycin RP-Mycin	Erythromicin
	Hosone	Erythromycin estolate
	E.E.S. E-Mycin E Pediamycin Wyamycin E	Erythromycin ethylsuccinate
	Ilotycin	Erythromycin gluceptate
	Erythrocin	Erythromycin lactobionate
	Bristamycin Erypar Erythrocin Ethril Pfizer-E SK-Erythromycin Wyamycin S	Erythromycin stearate

Continued.

Drugs or drug type	Brand names	Generic name
Estrogens (systemic)	TACE	Chlorotrianisene
	DES Stilphostrol	Diethylstilbestrol
	Delestrogen Estrace Progynon	Estradiol
	Premarin	Conjugated estrogens
	Amnestrogen	Esterified estrogens
	Theelin	Estrone
	Ogen Piperazine Estrone Sulfate	Estropipate
	Estinyl Feminone	Ethinyl estradiol
	Estrovis	Quinestrol
Estrogens (vaginal)	DV Cream	Dienestrol
	DES	Diethylstilbestrol
	Premarin	Conjugated estrogens
	Ogen Piperazine Estrone Sulfate	Estropipate
Estrogens and progestins—oral contraceptives (systemic)	Demulen	Ethynodiol diacetate and ethinyl estradiol
	Ovulen	Ethynodiol diacetate and mestranol
	Ovcon Brevicon Modicon	Norethindrone and ethinyl estradiol
	Norinyl Ortho-Novum	Norethindrone and mestranol
	Norlestrin Loestrin	Norethindrone acetate and ethinyl estradiol

Drugs or drug type	Brand names	Generic name
Estrogens and progestins—oral contraceptives (systemic)—cont'd	Enovid	Norethynodrel and mestranol
	Ovral Lo-Ovral	Norgestrel and ethinyl estradiol
Ethacrynic acid (systemic)	Edecrin	Ethacrynic acid
Ethambutol (systemic)	Myambutol	Ethambutol
Ethchlorvynol (systemic)	Placidyl	Ethchlorvynol
Ethinamate (systemic)	Valmid	Ethinamate
Ethionamide (systemic)	Trecator-SC	Ethionamide
Ethylnorepinephrine (systemic)	Bronkephrine	Ethylnorepinephrine
Fenfluramine (systemic)	Pondimin	Fenfluramine
Fenoprofen (systemic)	Nalfon	Fenoprofen
Flucytosine (systemic)	Ancobon	Flucytosine
Fluorouracil (systemic)	Adrucil	Fluorouracil
Furosemide (systemic)	Lasix Neo-renal	Furosemide
Gentian violet (vaginal)	Genapax Hyva	Gentian violet
Glutethimide (systemic)	Doriden Dormtabs	Glutethimide
Glycerin (systemic)	Glyrol Osmoglyn	
Griseofulvin (systemic)	Fulvicin P/G Fulvicin-U/F Grifulvin V Grisactin grisOwen Gris-PEG	Griseofulvin
Guaifenesin (systemic)	2/G Anti-Tuss	Guaifenesin

Continued.

Drugs or drug type	Brand names	Generic name
Guanifensin (systemic) —cont'd	Breonesin Genetuss Glycotuss Glytuss Hytuss Malotuss Nortussin Proco Robitussin	
Guaifenesin and codeine (systemic)	Cheracol Nortussin w/Codeine Robitussin A-C Tolu-Sed	
Guaifenesin and dextromethorphan (systemic)	Anti-Tuss DM Cheracol D Dextro-Tuss GG 2 G-DM G-Tuss DM Guaiadex Neo-Vadrin Queltuss Robitussin-DM Silexin Tolu-Sed DM Trocal Unproco	
Guanethidine (systemic)	Ismelin	Guanethidine
Guanethidine and hydrochlorothiazide (systemic)	Esimil	
Haloperidol (systemic)	Haldol	Haloperidol
Heparin (systemic)	Heprinar Lipo-Hepin Liquaemin Panheprin	Heparin
Hydantoin-type anticonvulsants (systemic)	Peganone	Ethotoin
	Mesantoin	Mephenytoin
	Dilantin Di-Phen Diphenylan Diphenylhydantoin	Phenytoin

Drugs or drug type	Brand names	Generic name
Hydralazine (systemic)	Apresoline	Hydralazine
Hydrocortisone (rectal)	Cortifoam Cort-Dome Proctocort	Hydrocortisone
Hydrocortisone, bismuth, benzyl benzoate, peruvian balsam, and zinc oxide (rectal)	Anusol-HC	
Hydroxyurea (systemic)	Hydrea	Hydroxyurea
Hydroxyzine (systemic)	Atarax Vistaril	Hydroxyzine
Ibuprofen (systemic)	Motrin	Ibuprofen
Indomethacin (systemic)	Indocin	Indomethacin
Insulin (systemic)	Actrapid Regular Insulin Regular Iletin II (new) Velosulin	Insulin injection
	Globin Insulin	Globin zinc insulin injection
	Insulatard NPH NPH Iletin II	Isophane insulin suspension
	Mixtard	Isophane insulin suspension and insulin injection
	Lentard Lente Insulin Lente Iletin II Monotard	Insulin zinc suspension
	Ultralente Ultralente Iletin Ultratard	Extended insulin zinc suspension
	Semilente Semilente Iletin Semitard	Prompt insulin zinc suspension

Continued.

Drugs or drug type	Brand names	Generic name
Insulin (systemic) —cont'd	Protamine Zinc & Iletin II PZI	Protamine zinc insulin suspension
Iodoquinol (systemic)	Moebiquin Yodoxin	Iodoquinol
Isoetharine (systemic)	Bronkometer Bronkosol	Isoetharine
Isometheptene, dichloralphenazone, and acetaminophen (systemic)	Midrin	
Isoniazid (systemic)	INH Nydrazid	Isoniazid
Isoproterenol (systemic)	Aerolone Iprenol Isuprel Medihaler-Iso Norisodrine Aerotrol Proternol Vapo-Iso	Isoproterenol
Isoproterenol and phenylephrine (systemic)	Duo-Medihaler	
Isoxsuprine (systemic)	Vasodilan Vasoprine	Isoxsuprine
Kanamycin (oral)	Kantrex	Kanamycin
Kaolin and pectin (oral)	Kaomead Kaopectate Pargel	
Kaolin, pectin, belladonna alkaloids, and opium (systemic)	Donnagel-PG	
Kaolin, pectin, and paregoric (systemic)	Parepectolin	
Laxatives, bulk-forming (oral)	Maltsupex Cellothyl	Malt soup extract Methylcellulose

Drugs or drug type	Brand names	Generic name
Laxatives, bulk-forming (oral)—cont'd	Cologel Hydrolose	
		Polycarbophil
	Mitrolan	Polycarbophil calcium
	Effersyllium Konsyl L.A. Formula Metamucil Modane Bulk Mucilose Plova Serutan Siblin	Psyllium mucilloid Psyllium seed Psyllium
Laxatives, emollient (oral)	Surfak	Docusate calcium
	Kasof	Docusate potassium
	Afko-Lube Colace Colax Comfolax Dioctyl Sodium Sulfo-succinate	Docusate sodium
	Alaxin Magcyl	Poloxamer 188
Laxatives, hyperosmotic-lactulose and saline (oral)	Chronulac	Lactulose
	Citrate of Magnesia	Magnesium citrate
	Adlerika Epsom Salt	Magnesium sulfate
	Phospho-Soda Sal Hepatica	Sodium phosphate (or phosphates) Effervescent sodium phosphate
Laxatives, lubricant (oral)	Liquid Petrolatum Nujol	Mineral oil
	Neo-Cultol	Mineral oil (jellied)
Laxatives, stimulant (oral)	Cenalax Codylax Dulcolax Theralax	Bisacodyl

Continued.

Drugs or drug type	Brand names	Generic name
Laxatives, stimulant (oral)—cont'd	Cascara Sagrada Cas-Evac	Cascara
	Alphamul Neoloid	Castor oil
	Dorbane Modane	Danthron
	Cholan-DH Decholin Neocholan	Dehydrocholic acid
	Alophen Espotabs Evac-U-Gen Evac-U-Lax Ex-Lax Feen-A-Mint Phenolax Prulet	Phenolphthalein
	Black Draught Casa Fru Dr. Caldwell's Senna Laxative Fletcher's Castoria Senokot Swiss Kriss X-Prep	Senna
	Glysennid Senokot X-Prep	Sennosides A and B
Levodopa (systemic)	Sinemet	Carbidopa and levodopa
	Bendopa Dopar Larodopa	Levodopa
Lincomycins (systemic)	Cleocin	Clindamycin
	Lincocin	Lincomycin
Lindane (topical)	Kwell	Lindane
Lithium (systemic)	Eskalith Lithonate	Lithium carbonate

Drugs or drug type	Brand names	Generic name
Lithium (systemic) —cont'd	Lithobid Lithonate-S Lithane	
Loperamide (systemic)	Imodium	Loperamide
Loxapine (systemic)	Daxolin Loxitane	Loxapine
Magnesia, milk of (oral)	Magnesia Magnesium hydroxide	
Mechlorethamine (systemic)	Mustargen	Mechlorethamine
Meclizine (systemic)	Bucladin-S	Buclizine
	Marezine	Cyclizine
	Antivert Bonine	Meclizine
Meclofenamate (systemic)	Meclomen	Meclofenamate
Melphalan (systemic)	Alkeran	Melphalan
Meperidine (systemic)	Demerol Pethadol	Meperidine
Meprobamate (systemic)	Equanil Meprospan Miltown SK-Bamate Tranmap	Meprobamate
Meprobamate, ethoheptazine, and aspirin (systemic)	Equagesic Heptogesic Mepro Compound Meprogesic	
Mercaptopurine (systemic)	Purinethol	Mercaptopurine
Metaproterenol (systemic)	Alupent Metaprel	Metaproterenol
Methadone (systemic)	Dolophine Westadone	Methadone

Continued.

Drugs or drug type	Brand names	Generic name
Methaqualone (systemic)	Mequin Parest Quaalude Sopor	Methaqualone
Methenamine (systemic)	Hiprex Urex	Methenamine hippurate
	Mandelamine Prov-U-Sep	Methenamine mandelate
Methocarbamol (systemic)	Delaxin Forbaxin Marbaxin-750 Metho-500 Robamol Robaxin Spinaxin Tumol	Methocarbamol
Methotrexate (systemic)	Mexate	Methotrexate
Methoxsalen (systemic)	Oxsoralen	Methoxsalen
Methyldopa (systemic)	Aldomet	Methyldopa
Methyldopa and thiazide diuretics (systemic)	Aldoclor	Methyldopa and chlorothiazide
	Aldoril	Methyldopa and hydro-chlorothiazide
Methylphenidate (systemic)	Ritalin	Methylphenidate
Methyprylon (systemic)	Noludar	Methyprylon
Methysergide (systemic)	Sansert	Methysergide
Metronidazole (systemic)	Flagyl	Metronidazole
Metyrosine (systemic)	Demser	Metyrosine
Miconazole (systemic)	Monistat	Miconazole
Miconazole (topical)	Micatin	Miconazole
Miconazole (vaginal)	Monistat	Miconazole

Drugs or drug type	Brand names	Generic name
Minoxidil (systemic)	Loniten	Minoxidil
Mithramycin (systemic)	Mithracin	Mithramycin
Mitomycin (systemic)	Mutamycin	Mitomycin
Mitotane (systemic)	Lysodren	Mitotane
Monoamine oxidase (MAO) inhibitors (systemic)	Marplan	Isocarboxazid
	Nardil	Phenelzine
	Parnate	Tranylcypromine
Nalbuphine (systemic)	Nubain	Nalbuphine
Nalidixic acid (systemic)	Neg Gram	Nalidixic acid
Naproxen (systemic)	Anaprox Naprosyn	Naproxen
Neomycin (oral)	Mycifradin Neobiotic	Neomycin
Neomycin, polymyxin B, and bacitracin (topical)	Mycitracin Neo-Polycin Neosporin	
Neomycin, polymyxin B, and gramicidin (ophthalmic)	Neo-Polycin Neosporin	
Nicotinyl alcohol (systemic)	Roniacol	Nicotinyl alcohol
Organic nitrates (other than nitroglycerin) (systemic)	Cardilate	Erythrityl tetranitrate
	Dilatrate-SR Iso-Bid Isordil Isotrate Sorate Sorbide Sorbitrate	Isosorbide dinitrate
	Duotrate Kaytrate Pentraspan Pentritol Peritrate	Pentaerythritol tetranitrate

Continued.

Drugs or drug type	Brand names	Generic name
Nitrofurantoin (systemic)	Cyantin Furadantin Macrodantin	
Nitroglycerin (systemic)	Glyceryl trinitrate Nitro-Bid Nitroglyn Nitrol Nitrong Nitrospan Nitrostat	Nitroglycerin
Nylidrin (systemic)	Arlidin	Nylidrin
Nystatin (oral)	Mycostatin Nilstat	Nystatin
Nystatin (topical)	Candex Mycostatin Nilstat	Nystatin
Nystatin (vaginal)	Korostatin Mycostatin Nilstat	Nystatin
Nystatin, neomycin, gramicidin, and triamcinolone (topical)	Mycolog Myco Triacet Mytrex Triamcinolone NNG	
Orphenadrine (systemic)	Flexojet Flexon Marflex Myolin Neocyten Norflex Ro-Orphena Tega-Flex X-Otag	
Orphenadrine and APC (systemic)	Norgesic Norgesic Forte	
Oxolinic acid (systemic)	Utibid	Oxolinic acid
Oxtriphylline and guaifenesin (systemic)	Brondecon Brondelate	

Drugs or drug type	Brand names	Generic name
Oxycodone and acetaminophen (systemic)	Percocet-5 Tylox	
Oxycodone and aspirin (systemic)	Percodan Percodan-Demi	
Oxymetazoline (nasal)	Afrin Duration St. Joseph Decongestant for Children	Oxymetazoline
Papaverine (systemic)	Cerebid Cerespan Dipav Dylate Hyobid Kavrin Myobid Orapav P-A-V Pavabid Pavacap Pavacon Pavadur Pavakey Pavased Pavasule Pavatest Pavatran Paverolan Ro-Papav Sustaverine Vasal Vasospan	Papaverine
Paraldehyde (systemic)	Paral	
Pargyline (systemic)	Eutonyl	
Pemoline (systemic)	Cylert	
Penicillamine (systemic)	Cuprimine Depen	
Penicillins (systemic)	Amoxil Larotid Polymox Robamox Sumox	Amoxicillin

Continued.

Drugs or drug type	Brand names	Generic name
Penicillins (systemic) —cont'd	Trimox	
	Utimox	
	Wymox	
	Amcill	Ampicillin
	Omnipen	
	Penbritin	
	Pensyn	
	Polycillin	
	Principen	
	Supen	
	Totacillin	
	Geocillin	Carbenicillin
	Geopen	
	Pyopen	
	Cloxapen	Cloxacillin
	Tegopen	
	Cyclapen-W	Cyclacillin
	Dycill	Dicloxacillin
	Dynapen	
	Pathocil	
	Veracillin	
	Versapen	Hetacillin
	Versapen-K	
	Azapen	Methicillin
	Celbenin	
	Staphcillin	
	Nafcil	Nafcillin
	Unipen	
	Bactocill	Oxacillin
	Prostaphlin	
	Bicillin	Penicillin G
	Crysticillin	
	Duracillin	
	Pentids	
	Permapen	
	Wycillin	
	Betapen-VK	Penicillin V
	Penapar VK	
	Pen-Vee K	

Drugs or drug type	Brand names	Generic name
Penicillins (systemic) —cont'd	Uticillin VK V-Cillin Veetids	
	Ticar	Ticarcillin
Pentazocine (systemic)	Talwin	Pentazocine
Pentazocine and aspirin (systemic)	Talwin Compound	
Pentobarbital and carbromal (systemic)	Carbrital	
Perphenazine and amitriptyline (systemic)	Etrafon Triavil	
Phenazopyridine (systemic)	Azo-100 Azodine Azo-Standard Di-Azo Phen-Azo Phenazodine Pyridiate Pyridium Pyrodine	Phenazopyridine
Phenothiazines (systemic)	Tindal	Acetophenazine
	Repoise	Butaperizine
	Proketazine	Carphenazine
	Chloramead Promapar Thorazine	Chlorpromazine
	Permitil Prolixin	Fluphenazine
	Serentil	Mesoridazine
	Trilafon	Perphenazine
	Quide	Piperacetazine
	Compazine Stemetil	Prochlorperazine

Continued.

Drugs or drug type	Brand names	Generic name
Phenothiazines (systemic)—cont'd	Sparine	Promazine
	Mellaril	Thioridazine
	Stelazine	Trifluoperazine
	Vesprin	Triflupromazine
Phenoxybenzamine	Dibenzyline	
Phenylbutazone (systemic)	Oxalid Tandearil	Oxyphenbutazone
	Azolid Butazolidin	Phenylbutazone
	Azolid-A Butazolidin Alka Phenylzone-A	Buffered phenylbutazone
Phenylephrine (nasal)	Alcon-Efrin Allerest Contac Coricidin Isophrin Neo-Mist Neo-Synephrine Pyracort-D Rhinall Sinarest Super Anahist Synasal Vacon	
Phenylpropanolamine (systemic)	Coffee-Break Control Delcopro Diadax Dietac Obestat Pro-Dax 21 Propadrine Rhindecon	
Phenylpropanolamine, phenylephrine, phenyltoloxamine, and chlorpheniramine (systemic)	Naldecon	
Potassium iodide (systemic)	K1-N Pima	Potassium iodide

Drugs or drug type	Brand names	Generic name
Potassium phosphates (systemic)	K-Phos Original	Monobasic potassium phosphates
	Neutra-Phos-K	Potassium phosphates
Potassium and sodium phosphates (systemic)	Uro-KP-Neutral	Dibasic potassium and sodium phosphates
	K-Phos M. F. K-Phos Neutral K-Phos No. 2	Monobasic potassium and sodium phosphates
	Neutra-Phos	Potassium and sodium phosphates
Potassium supplements (systemic)	Potassium Triplex Tri-K Trikates	Potassium acetate, potassium bicarbonate, and potassium citrate
	K-Lyte	Potassium bicarbonate and citric acid
	KEFF	Potassium bicarbonate, potassium carbonate, and potassium chloride
	Klorvess	Potassium bicarbonate and potassium chloride
	K-Lyte/Cl	Potassium bicarbonate, potassium chloride, and citric acid
	Kaochlor-Eff	Potassium bicarbonate, potassium chloride, and potassium citrate
	Kaochlor Kaon-Cl Kato Kay-Ciel K-Lor KLOR-10% KLOR-CON Klorvess Klotrix K-Lyte/Cl Slow-K	Potassium chloride
	Kolyum	Potassium chloride and potassium gluconate

Continued.

Drugs or drug type	Brand names	Generic name
Potassium supplements (systemic)—cont'd	Twin-K	Potassium citrate and potassium gluconate
	Kaon	Potassium gluconate
Prazosin (systemic)	Minipress	Prazosin
Primidone (systemic)	Mysoline	Primidone
Probenecid (systemic)	Benemid Probalan	Probenecid
Probucol (systemic)	Lorelco	Probucol
Procainamide (systemic)	Procamide Procan Procan SR Procopan Pronestyl Sub-Quin	Procainamide
Procarbazine (systemic)	Matulane	Procarbazine
Prochlorperazine and isopropamide (systemic)	Combid	
Progestins (systemic)	Duphaston	Dydrogesterone
	Delalutin	Hydroxyprogesterone
	Provera	Medroxyprogesterone
	Megace	Megestrol
	Micronor Nor-Q.D. Norlutin	Norethindrone
	Norlutate	Norethindrone acetate
	Ovrette	Norgestrel
	Proluton Lipo-Lutin	Progesterone
Promethazine (systemic)	Historest Phenergan Remsed	Promethazine

Drugs or drug type	Brand names	Generic name
Propantheline (systemic)	Pro-Banthine	Propantheline
Propoxyphene (systemic)	Darvon Dolene Pargesic 65 Proxagesic Proxene SK-65	Propoxyphene
Propoxyphene and acetaminophen (systemic)	Darvocet-N Dolacet Dolene AP-65 SK-65-APAP Wygesic	
Propoxyphene and APC (systemic)	Darvon Compound Dolene Compound-65 SK-65 Compound	
Propoxyphene and aspirin (systemic)	Darvon with A.S.A. Darvon-N with A.S.A.	
Pseudoephedrine (systemic)	Afrinol D-Feda Neobid Novafed Ro-Fedrin Sudafed Sudrin	Pseudoephedrine
Pyrilamine and pentobarbital (systemic)	Eme-Nil Wans	
Pyrithione zinc (topical)	Danex Head and Shoulders Zincon	
Pyrvinium (systemic)	Povan	Pyrvinium
Quinidine (systemic)	Cardioquin Cin-Quin Duraquin Quinaglute Dura-Tabs Quinidex Extentabs Quinora	
Quinine (systemic)	Coco-Quinine Quine	Quinine

Continued.

Drugs or drug type	Brand names	Generic name
Quinine and aminophylline (systemic)	Quinamm Quinite Strema	
Rauwolfia alkaloids (systemic)	Harmonyl	Deserpidine
	Raudixin	
	Raulfia Raupoid Rauserpa	Rauwolfia serpentina
	Rau-Sed Reserpoid Sandril Serpasil	Reserpine
Rauwolfia alkaloids and thiazide diuretics (systemic)	Oreticyl Oreticyl Forte	Deserpidine and hydrochlorothiazide
	Enduronyl	Deserpidine and methyclothiazide
	Rauzide	Rauwolfia serpentina and bendroflumethiazide
	Exna-R	Reserpine and benzthiazide
	Diupres	Reserpine and chlorothiazide
	Demi-Regroton Regroton	Reserpine and chlorthalidone
	Hydropres Reserpazide Serpasil-Esidrix	Reserpine and hydrochlorothiazide
	Salutensin Salutensin-Demi	Reserpine and hydroflumethiazide
	Diutensen-R	Reserpine and methylclothiazide
	Renese-R	Reserpine and polythiazide
	Hydromox-R	Reserpine and quinethazone

Drugs or drug type	Brand names	Generic name
Rauwolfa alkaloids and thiazide diuretics (systemic)—cont'd	Metatensin Naquival	Reserpine and trichlormethiazide
Reserpine and hydralazine (systemic)	Serpasil-Apresoline	
Reserpine, hydralazine, and hydrochlorothiazide (systemic)	Ser-Ap-Es Tri-Hydroserpine	
Resorcinol and sulfur (topical)	Acne-Dome Acnomel Cenac Exzit pHisoAc Sulforcin	
Rifampin (systemic)	Rifadin Rimactane	Rifampin
Rifampin and isoniazid (systemic)	Rifamate	
Salicyclates (systemic)	Bayer Aspirin Ecotrin Empirin Analgesic Measurin St. Joseph Aspirin	Aspirin
	Ascriptin Bufferin CAMA Inlay-Tabs	Buffered aspirin
	Calurin	Carbaspirin
	Arthropan	Choline salicylate
	Parbocyl Uracel	Sodium salicylate
Salicylic acid and sulfur (topical)	Acne-Dome Acno Antiseb BUF Exzit Fostex Klaron Meted Pernox Rezamid	

Continued.

Drugs or drug type	Brand names	Generic name
Salicylic acid and sulfur (topical)—cont'd	SAStid Sebex Sebulex Therac Vanseb	
Salicylic acid, sulfur, and coal tar (topical)	Antiseb-T Sebex-T Sebutone Vanseb-T	
Selenium sulfide (topical)	Exsel Iosel Selsun Selsun Blue Sul-Blue	
Sodium fluoride (systemic)	Denta-Fl Flo-Tab Fluorident Fluoritab Fluorodex Flura Karidium Luride Luride-SF Nafeen Pedi-Dent Pediaflor Stay-Flo Studaflor	
Spironolactone (systemic)	Aldactone	Spironolactone
Spironolactone and hydrochlorothiazide (systemic)	Aldactazide	
Succinimide-type anticonvulsants (systemic)	Zarontin Celontin Milontin Ethosuximide Methsuximide Phensuximide	
Sulfasalazine (systemic)	Azulfidine S.A.S.-500	Sulfasalazine
Sulfinpyrazone (systemic)	Anturane Zynol	Sulfinpyrazone

Drugs or drug type	Brand names	Generic name
Sulfonamides (systemic)	Renoquid	Sulfacytine
	Gantanol Methoxal Methoxanol	Sulfamethoxazole
	Bactrim Septra	Sulfamethoxazole and trimethoprim
	Gantrisin Lipo Gantrisin Sosol Sulfalar Sulfizin	Sulfisoxazole
Sulfonamides (vaginal)	AVC Femguard Nil Tricholan Vagidine Vagimine Vagitrol	Sulfanilamide, aminacrine, and allantoin
	Sultrin Trysul	Sulfathiazole, sulfacetamide, and sulfabenzamide
	Koro-Sulf	Sulfisoxazole
	Vagilia	Sulfisoxazole, aminacrine, and allantoin
Sulfonamides and phenazopyridine (systemic)	Azo Gantanol	Sulfamethoxazole and phenazopyridine
	Azo Gantrisin Azo-Soxazole Azosul Azo-Sulfizin Suldiazo	Sulfisoxazole and phenazopyridine
Sulindac (systemic)	Clinoril	Sulindac
Tamoxifen (systemic)	Nolvadex	Tamoxifen
Terbutaline (systemic)	Brethine Bricanyl	Terbutaline
Terpin hydrate and codeine (systemic)	Cortussis	

Continued.

Drugs or drug type	Brand names	Generic name
Testolactone (systemic)	Teslac	Testolactone
Tetracyclines (systemic)	Declomycin	Demeclocycline
	Doxychel Doxy-Tabs Vibramycin Vibra-Tabs	Doxycycline
	Rondomycin	Methacycline
	Minocin	Minocycline
	Oxlopar Oxy-Kesso-Tetra Terramycin Tetramine	Oxytetracycline
	Achromycin Bristacycline Cyclopar Panmycin Retet Robitet Sumycin Tetracyn	Tetracycline
Theophylline, ephedrine, and barbiturates (systemic)	Asminyl Asma-lief Phedral Tedfern Tedral Thalfed Thedrizem Theodrine Theofed Theofenal Theoral Theotabs	
Theophylline, ephedrine, guaifenesin, and barbiturates (systemic)	Broncholate Bronkolixir Bronkotabs Duovent Luftodil Mudrane GG Quibron Plus Verequad	

Drugs or drug type	Brand names	Generic name
Theophylline, ephedrine, and hydroxyzine (systemic)	Asminorel	
	E.T.H. Compound	
	Hydrophed	
	Marax	
	Theophozine	
	Theozine	
Theophylline and guaifenesin (systemic)	Asbron G	
	Asma	
	Cerylin	
	Dialixir	
	Glybron	
	Glyceryl T	
	Hylate	
	Lanophyllin-GG	
	Quibron	
	Slo-Phyllin GG	
	Synophylate-GG	
	Theo-Col	
	Theo-Guaia	
Thiazide diuretics (systemic)	Naturetin	Bendroflumethiazide
	Aquastat	Benzthiazide
	Aquatag	
	Exna	
	Hydrex	
	Diuril	Chlorothiazide
	SK-Chlorothiazide	
	Hygroton	Chlorthalidone
	Uridon	
	Anhydron	Cyclothiazide
	Esidrix	Hydrochlorothiazide
	Hydro-Aquil	
	HydroDIURIL	
	Oretic	
	Diucardin	Hydroflumethiazide
	Saluron	
	Aquatensen	Methyclothiazide
	Duretic	
	Enduron	
	Diulo	Metolazone
	Zaroxolyn	

Continued.

Drugs or drug type	Brand names	Generic name
Thiazide diuretics (systemic)—cont'd	Renese	Polythiazide
	Hydromox	Quinethazone
	Metahydrin Naqua	Trichlormethiazide
Thioxanthenes (systemic)	Taractan	Chlorprothixene
	Navane	Thiothixene
Thyroid hormones (systemic)	Levothroid L-T-S Ro-Thyroxine Synthroid	Levothyroxine
	Cytomel Ro-Thyronine Tertroxin	Liothyronine
	Euthroid	Liotrix
	Proloid	Thyroglobulin
	S-P-T Thyrar Thyrocrine	Thyroid
Thyrotropin (systemic)	Thyrotron Thytropar	Thyrotropin
Tolmetin (systemic)	Tolectin	Tolmetin
Tolnaftate (topical)	Aftate Tinactin	Tolnaftate
Tretinoin (topical)	Retin-A	Tretinoin
Triamterene (systemic)	Dyrenium	Triamterene
Triamterene and hydrochlorothiazide (systemic)	Dyazide	
Tricyclic antidepressants (systemic)	Amitid Amitil Elavil Endep	Amitriptyline
	Norpramin Pertofrane	Desipramine

Drugs or drug type	Brand names	Generic name
Tricyclic antidepressants (systemic)—cont'd	Adapin Sinequan	Doxepin
	Imavate Janimine SK-Pramine Tofranil	Imipramine
	Aventyl Pamelor	Nortriptyline
	Vivactil	Protriptyline
	Surmontil	Trimipramine
Trimethobenzamide (systemic)	Tigan	Trimethobenzamide
Triprolidine and pseudoephedrine (systemic)	Actifed Allerphed Tagafed	
Undecylenic acid, compound (topical)	Decylenes Desenex Medaped Quinsana Plus	
Urea (systemic)	Ureaphil	
Valproic acid (systemic)	Depakene	Valproic acid
Vinblastine (systemic)	Velban	Vinblastine
Vincristine (systemic)	Oncovin	Vincristine
Vitamins and fluoride (systemic)	Vita-Flor Adeflor Mulvidren-F Novacebrin with Fluoride Vi-Penta F Poly-Vi-Flor V-Daylin with Fluoride	Multiple vitamins and fluoride
	Cari-Tab Tri-Vi-Flor	Vitamins A, D, and C and fluoride

Continued.

Drugs or drug type	Brand names	Generic name
(methyl)-Xanthines (systemic)	Aminodur Lixaminol Mini-Lix Somophyllin	Aminophylline
	Airet Dilin Dilor Lufyllin Neothylline	Dyphylline
	Choledyl	Oxtriphylline
	Accurbron Aerolate Bronkodyl Elixicon Elixophyllin Physpan Slophyllin Somophyllin-T Theobid Theoclear Theodur Theolair Theolixir Theophyl Theospan	Theophylline
Xylometazoline (nasal)	4-Way Long Acting Neo-Synephrine II Otrivin Rhinall Long Acting Sine-Off Once-A-Day Sinex Long-Acting Sinutab Long Acting Sinus Spray	

Index

T

U

V

W

X

Y

Z